The Forgivers Club
Where You Can Be Dead Honest...

by

L.W. Hawksby

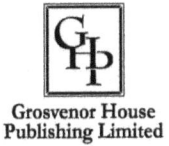

Grosvenor House
Publishing Limited

All rights reserved
Copyright © L.W. Hawksby, 2021

The right of L.W. Hawksby to be identified as the author of this
work has been asserted in accordance with Section 78
of the Copyright, Designs and Patents Act 1988

The book cover is copyright to L.W. Hawksby

This book is published by
Grosvenor House Publishing Ltd
Link House
140 The Broadway, Tolworth, Surrey, KT6 7HT.
www.grosvenorhousepublishing.co.uk

This book is sold subject to the conditions that it shall not, by way of
trade or otherwise, be lent, resold, hired out or otherwise circulated
without the author's or publisher's prior consent in any form of binding or
cover other than that in which it is published and
without a similar condition including this condition being imposed
on the subsequent purchaser.

This book is a work of fiction. Any resemblance to
people or events, past or present, is purely coincidental.

A CIP record for this book
is available from the British Library

ISBN 978-1-83975-510-1

Dedicated to Kyle; the man who saw me go to Hell and tried, more than anyone, to bring me home.

Disclaimer and Author's Note

The Forgivers Club is my third book and second novel. Like my previous works, this story has a lot of elements that you will find triggering and shocking. As an author, I choose to focus on writing about criminality and the many ways it can seem to "come out of nowhere" and impact the lives around the person acting that way. Few people understand or even care that, in the face of extreme distress, pain or even *in victimhood*, a broken person can end up doing something awful and gaining the label of "Criminal".

I have made extra efforts to alter names and other defining characteristics in this book, to such an extent that I hope it will be enjoyed as fiction, although it was inspired by true events.

The *biggest* changes I have made to protect the anonymity of the characters involved include locating "The Forgivers Club" in a different country, giving the village a fictional name, altering names. I have also changed many of the lead characters' defining characteristics, to anonymise the people our heroine engages with in the book.

This book was not written and released to cause anyone any distress. This book, like my others, was written to explore taboo subjects and to make people think about common (yet rarely exposed) issues such as vigilantism, journalistic harassment, and the terrible power of abusive friendships. I also wanted to write about how a person's sexual identity and decision-making can be warped by *bullying, dark tetrad personality disorder abuse, betrayal trauma* and *domestic violence.* Unfortunately, that outcome is not rare, and neither is it fiction.

As ever, I hope my writing will, in some way, make the world a more just and safer place, for everyone.

Contents

Prologue	ix
Chapter 1: Merry Christmas Baby	1
Chapter 2: Running Water	11
Chapter 3: Bridgefell	17
Chapter 4: Dirty, Dirty Men!	40
Chapter 5: White Water	48
Chapter 6: Filth	57
Chapter 7: The Mistake	67
Chapter 8: The Drowning	81
Chapter 9: Green-eyed	95
Chapter 10: Perfect	103
Chapter 11: A Woman Scorned	110
Chapter 12: Trapped	122
Chapter 13: Beaten Down	126
Chapter 14: Warnings	139
Chapter 15: Burnt	147
Chapter 16: She Said, She Said	153
Chapter 17: Trapped Again	159
Chapter 18: The Island	170
Chapter 19: Rattling	179
Chapter 20: A Hiding	193
Chapter 21: She's Dead	201
Chapter 22: Guilty Party	207
Epilogue	219

*****

Prologue

As the kicks rain down one by one, a thought skitters by and stops - a forgotten leaf on the wind, caught on a coat collar – *I'm going to die here tonight. Laid on this cold wet pavement with these boots and shoes and trainers pounding me and not a soul will care. Maybe no one will even know. I'm all alone in this place, a place I came to for safety.*

Someone's grunting and swearing; calling me obscene names punctuating each kick. I've given up trying to fight them off. No point. There's three of them, maybe more will join in. Looking up, I can see puffs of frozen air as they breathe, each one giving them more energy to continue their beating. The coldness is seeping through my clothes. There are no stars tonight and, even if there were, they would be hiding behind my attackers, as they bend over me, close together as if in a rugby scrum.

Moving my head in an attempt to evade the blows to my face, I can feel my hair's been pulled out of the pretty Heidi-plaits I wove earlier, in anticipation of a fun night out with friends. That seems so long ago now, and I know I was so wrong to trust anyone, to dare think I could have a normal life here.

A kick to the side of my face makes me cry out but I'm soon distracted by another in my right rib, swiftly followed by one to my right thigh. The pulling and tugging makes me think of what it must be like to be dragged by demons to Hell.

It's all in slow-motion; the body's way of protecting the mind from the terror while still saving as much detail as possible. I close my eyes and give in to the brutality, waiting for that one special blow that will shut me down. For good.

Barking in the distance. A whooshing, sucking feeling, and then every detail and sound sharpens in focus, as though jolted awake from a nightmare. Present in the moment again, I taste blood.

Flickering into life, I kick out. *That's Phoebe!* She's scared. Barking and howling, louder now. She yaps and wails over and over. *I'm not alone.* Not at all. So much noise, and then a rush of pure fear. Perfectly-timed adrenalin. Now I'm fucked off. *Fuck this!* I'm not leaving my baby in this place. This evil terrible place with these monsters.

Drawing my knees up, I kick out. Both legs. Both feet. Bang! Left then right, I get two of my attackers. My skinny PVC-wrapped legs and my feet, big for someone who's 48 kilos and only 5'4, are pretty strong. I catch one on the shin, another on the knee. It's a sickening yet satisfying release of sound. Again, I kick out but I miss. They've stepped back a little yet are still aiming for my ribs and head, with great force. Gaining in anger and bravery, I dare to reach up and to grab an arm, or a sleeve. The kicks are still coming but I've stopped feeling them; focused entirely on getting up, I've found the sleeve or maybe the hem of one of my attackers' coat. I pull hard and they fall forward.

Leveraging their weight, I've found my own feet again, even in heels. My sudden defensive reaction to the beating has stunned them, the attack's stopped.

Standing in the middle of these three women, I'm panting, my head bent down a little but I'm looking straight ahead. Bull-like, horns down, I want to charge at them and kill them. Stamp on *their* heads. Gore them and kick *their* faces. Tear *their* clothes, like they did mine. Pull their hair, like they did to me.

My scalp is burning now, and I close my eyes in pain. The women use this moment of vulnerability to make their escape. They've done what they came for. They are bigger than me. Two are older. *Dear god!* Yes, now I know who they are.

"We need to go. She's seen us now. Our faces!" a husky, urgent voice behind me. Then they're gone. Running. Scattering in all directions. Birds flapping up and away. Startled by the sneak of a cat.

I'm more than happy to show claws. Risk yet another of my nine lives. Raising my fists and weaving slightly, one of my legs gives way. I'm too exhausted to run after them.

I watch as all three slide away into the oily night. Their footsteps grow fainter, but I hear their voices clammering and echoing together. In their panic, they've forgotten to stay anonymous. The light from a shop window illuminating the women for a brief second, shows me small details that scar my memory. A white T-shirt with flying birds over a large bust. A black jacket and black hair. An orange vest clashing with greying, orange hair.

Someone is looking out of a window across the street, and a person coming back from the corner shop has stopped dead on the other side of the road. No one comes to help me. And when they see me looking at them, both witnesses turn their heads away; one into their hood, the other ducking back behind a net curtain.

Taking a tentative step forward, nothing hurts but I'm stiff with shock. That scares me. I know what it feels like to be beaten; the pain, bruises, cuts and scars, come later.

Crying silently and limping now, because both shoes are damaged. Oh yeah, I can tell one is missing a heel. Now I am dreading looking at my reflection in the mirror, once I get home. I stagger down the street and hope to not be seen by anyone else, the opposite of any other attack victim. Chances are I will either be photographed and laughed at, or maybe even attacked again. Heading towards the shop where I used to work , I'm collecting Phoebe and leaving this treacherous, evil place.

The sounds of their escape fade, as the women disappear into the dark, helped by the rabbit warren of small narrow streets that circle the place I loved most in the world.

A nest of food, joy and hope that was supposed to be my safe place. A place to go to and heal from a relationship with the man who ruined me from the inside out. To escape both him and the woman who works with him stalking and harassing anyone she sees as a threat. I came here to escape their vile, toxic union.

Chapter 1: Merry Christmas Baby

I've felt it coming; all the signs are there. All the red flags a'waving. That sickness in my gut and that metallic taste of dread on my tongue. His afternoon naps, the slightly crazed look on his face when he thinks I'm not looking. Even his right pupil's bigger than the other - just like last time.

He's been moody for three days now; phone attached to his hand or comfortably out of sight. The small square outline visible through the tight fit of the arse pocket of his denims. The insect-like buzzing; message after message and call after call, making him walk away from me to another room, or to go to the toilet, for the 20th time that day.

He couldn't even keep it in his pants for fucking Christmas; our third Christmas. As if the last one wasn't bad enough?!

The disappearing act on New Year's Day and "accidental" leaving me on his mother's sofa to go home, while I slept off a night out on yet another empty stomach. I mean, who leaves their fiancée on their mother's sofa, six miles from home? *Jamie does.*

This year, he'll probably try and do it again; he likes to test his "escape acts" and finding new ways to spend time away from me to cheat, to take street drugs, and to groom new victims.

It's always my fault though; "You fell asleep. You drank too much".

"I've worked hard and need space from your constant nagging. I'm going to John's".

"I don't feel well. I think I'm going to relapse. I'm going to stay at mum's tonight. Being around you makes me ill".

I know Jamie's script as well as he does. My acting skills are improving, as I try to survive this snuff film, day after day.

He's big enough and ugly enough, with steroids and six trips to the gym each week, to have carried me to the car and taken me home like any normal, caring bloke would. But, of course, he left me at his mother's, to go back and see my friend. A fresh face and fresh meat opportunity who had happily joined our New Year's Eve party at a local Indian restaurant.

Jamie hadn't met her before, so to him she was an ideal feast. Her full round face, naïve little jokes and grinning as he brushed past her, or ogled her tits across the table.

Oh god, what an embarrassment! He got what he wanted, and she probably regretted it as soon as he left her bed; she wasn't his type to keep around. Too old. Too vocal. And as a friend of mine, far, far, too risky. I know Jamie prefers customers from his job at the Leisure Centre, so he was, how you say...? branching out, with a friend of mine. Again. He will have blocked and blanked her as he got in his car to drive home to shower, before coming to collect me.

So, this year, yet another year, I prayed it'd be different. Another 12 months has passed. Four more seasons and countless fake-apologies have spurted from his mouth or lit up my phone. Another year of even more adventurous, increasingly dark and rough sex. Another year, this time with three more relapses, two more detoxes and what felt like a million AA meetings. *All for nothing.* This time though, right here, right now, I feel different; detached and angry.

Stony-faced, I'm watching him play on that fucking phone and suck on his fake cigarette again and again. He flushes pink and gets sweaty every now and then, most likely at yet another disgusting picture he sends, or some stupid female sends him. Moving towards him triggers a flinch and the phone's turned face down and laid on his lap as he smiles tightly up at me. He lets me kiss or embrace him, but he returns the gesture with a stiffness I recognise as anger and discomfort, at being interrupted in his filthy exploits and being almost caught out... again.

I did this little manoeuvre just a few minutes ago; stood up suddenly to get another glass of wine. He nearly jumped out of his skin; scaly, nasty skin. I was too quick for him this time and caught the arousal-snarl on his lips and the big pink tits on the screen before he could react fast enough.

Bile rose in my throat as I poured the wine in my favourite glass; deep, almost black, red, I drank half the glass in one, to dilute the sick that was threatening to appear in my mouth.

Phoebe watches him too. Her fur is a barometer of my own rage and disgust towards the man she has never liked. A white Staffordshire Bull Terrier, she's small, plump, and heavy as hell. Intuitive and sensitive to any change in the atmosphere, it creates in her the subtle changes that I alone can read. The fluffy-fur thing means she knows I'm about to lose my temper, although it would be the first time with Jamie.

I've developed a terrible paranoia and temper around other people. Excessive, frightening and out of control, I take my fear and panic out on anyone I see as a threat to us. Jamie has worked his dark magic very skilfully.

I worry that I have become like Sharna, the woman obsessed with us breaking up so she can get her Devil back. The woman who has stalked and harassed me for the last few years, since I met Jamie and fell into what I thought was love. I don't fear her or anyone else. Not even the debts that I juggle. Not even the worry about the damage I'm doing to my body. Not even my parents dying of the illnesses that blight the last years of their lives. I am numb to anything but him. I fear nothing and no one, but him. It's the sickness of us; the toxicity of *this*.

Don't get me wrong, the violence isn't that common; it's only been four times. I can cope with that. The most recent time he hit me, I begged him to schedule in a slap and kick each morning before work, in exchange for no more cheating, drugging and lies.

Of course, he laughed in my face and I cried. Then he kissed me hard. Pushing his tongue into my mouth and keeping his eyes open to make sure I was reading his signals; the kiss and embrace his promise and gagging order, that all that week's upset was to be forgotten. As usual.

Last year, my periods stopped from the stress; he was delighted but I wasn't. He thought I was pregnant! So convinced by what a wonderful partner he was, it didn't cross his mind that the abuse had affected my body to such an extent. I knew it was impossible that I was expecting his baby; I'd simply lied to his face and pretended to come off my pill, unlike the other fools he's trapped in the past.

So, no "monthly" arrived and he made his assumptions and I let him make them! It was the first tiny semblance of control I had held in a long time.

Yes, I held that secret tight and close to me; a fat, proud and growing lie. The only secret I had from him, until now. The strange thing is, he wasn't disappointed when I didn't flower and bloom with his child in the following months. By the time it was obvious he had failed in his penile-mission, he was already focusing on some new project with white veiny breasts and a birth date too close to the age of consent.

Watching him from the doorway between kitchen and living-room, I know for a fact he just thinks he can keep trying; pumping away, spreading his seed when he likes, and adding to the cluster of disturbed and neglected children he already has. Children he barely sees or pays for. Small versions of him that he willingly planted, in three torn and fractured families scattered like bones over the city we are forced to share with them.

Removing myself - no disentangling myself - from the dragging, sucking tentacles of this relationship has taken time. I made the decision to plan my escape a few weeks ago. It's not just the signs of cheating again, it's what happened on Halloween this year. His rage and tantrum came out of nowhere and shocked me to the core. Why that time? Why was **that** the final straw? Because I hadn't seen it coming for once.

The change in behaviour and swing from slightly moody, to the torrential raining down of accusations and jealousy, took seconds. It's never been this bad before. It scared me and my lack of preparedness scared me too. I knew then that my lack of instinct was failing me as it does with so many of these *dangerous normal people,* these domestic abusers and people users.

* * * * * * * * * * * * * *

"I'm just walking in. Give me a second while I park the car! Make sure you're ready to leave straight away, 'coz I'm parked dodgy and it's getting busier with these fucking stupid trick or treaters, or whatever they're called!" Jamie is out of breath and sounds stressed. My gut clenches at this red flag for a drama and immediately I'm regretting my stupid silly surprise. He usually likes me to dress up, especially if it shows off my legs and slender body.

Before I can gather the words of apology like marbles in my mouth, he's striding through people, past the band, towards me. The crowd parts and my heart compresses in fear. "What the fuck do you think you're wearing!? You said you weren't going to dress up". He's hissing in my face and I'm dumbstruck at how obvious his rage is.

"I just got carried away with it all. The rest of the staff dressed up... and...". I flick my eyes towards the girl I work with, to see if she's noticed. There's no sign of her, but I hear her laughing around the corner. That's good. She's serving a customer at the other end of the large, curved bar.

She's been telling me to end this misery since I started working here. She doesn't understand that I'm waiting for him to get clean again, to go back to how he was when we met. When we were *perfect.*

"It's all so guys look at you, isn't it? You're so fucking needy. Same with all those selfies and gym pictures on Facebook", he whispers harshly. Spittle lands on my face. A few people close enough to hear look at us, but turn away in embarrassment.

My beloved partner has conveniently forgotten about his own constant social media presence, and that social media is his absolute favourite hunting and hurting ground.

"Jamie, it's just a bit of fun. I'll get changed as soon as we get home. I'll delete the pics I put on Facebook and on my works page…" My whining calms him. He steps back and smiles, looks around to see if anyone is watching then lifts me up off the floor and embraces me as though he's delighted with my Halloween costume, after all.

The short purple and black net skirt is crushed between us and he smears my face-paint. As he drops me back to the ground, I am a little broken doll and blush deeply in shame. "Let's go home, Jamie". I take his hand and lead him out of the pub, holding back the flood of tears I know will agitate him even more.

****

I didn't see it coming; the slap in the car park, pressed up against the wall by the bins.

Driving home, Jamie was silent. Seething. His jaw clenching and his face furious. His knuckles on the steering wheel were white and the coarse skin from his psoriasis, seemed to pulse with rage. I desperately needed the toilet; the fear of his rages had developed to such a high stage by then, I'd developed I.B.S. Even if he weren't violent, he'd be so cruel with his words and actions that the sense of dread when he kicked off felt worse than any slap or tight hands wrapped around my throat.

This time the slap was harder than before, aimed right at the side of my head rather than delicate skin on my face. My ear rang for a full day after it and, if I squeezed my eyes shut, the scalp felt tender enough to encourage a moan and yet more tears.

Of course, he'd wanted to make up in the early hours of the morning, his *usual* way. I just lay there and waited for him to finish. The final shreds of emotion I had for him were trapped around my wrists, as my pulse quickened in disgust. Although I felt trapped by twisted love, toxic attachment, and fear of repercussions, I knew I had to leave. He was escalating, and the sex felt more and more like rape.

It was after these times, as I cringed in disgust at his look of being well-fed after sex, that my thoughts turned to Sharna. How he will have treated her this same way; a blow-up doll with no feelings, and no loyalty to the other "dolls" he shared his sexual proclivities with. To have to sleep with someone you know has (and is continuing) to masturbate to a series of people on the internet, and fuck (unprotected) whoever he can get his grimy hands on, is *absolute torture*.

I knew better than to say no to his manhood prodding and poking in my lower back, grunting demands and rough hands on my breasts, tugging and pulling me backwards towards him.

I hear the bedroom door close shut quietly; he's away to masturbate and film it again. Closing my eyes and leaning against the kitchen counter in abject exhaustion, I fill my glass up again and remember.

The first time I denied Jamie was only a few months after we met, almost three years ago now. That dark path took me to terrible places. I hate thinking about it.

My lover's response that first time I wriggled away from him, explaining I was tired and stressed about my estranged husband's constant bullying, was to push me out of the bed.

Wearing only underwear, I was forced to sit in a corner while Jamie slept. "You don't want to share a bed with me properly, Lola? Well, you don't get to share a bed with me at all", he'd said. Jamie, as usual, ghosted and discarded me; he didn't speak to me for two days after it and I was told to go back to my own flat.

Why didn't I end it then? I can work that out once I've left. Once my brain can rest and my soul can sleep; I'll work it out then. For now, the most important thing is to *leave*.

Going back into the living room to tidy up and prepare for bed, I find him playing on his phone again, with an obvious erection through his favourite red shorts. So, silent, I return to the kitchen to carry on washing up from dinner. Numb to it now, finally, I have a plan of action that for the first time in a long time has me ever so slightly positive about the future.

It's Christmas Day tomorrow and my gift to myself has come early; that shiny, sparkling gem of an idea to escape in the early hours, while he sleeps.

"Lola?! Baby?! Can you bring me a can in?" Jamie is drinking again, although in all honesty not as heavily as AA says addicts in relapse do. His real addiction is drugs, it's easier for him to hide that from the "fans" he has wiggling their saggy boobs and slobbering all over him in the NA and AA groups he likes to cruise for victims.

I sound so bitter! And I really am! Hateful and bitter... not sweet and naïve like I used to be, before he and Sharna entered my life and set fire to it.

"Lola?! Are you coming in and bringing me a drink or not?!" Jamie sounds exasperated, and my pulse quickens in fear. I need to leave before he discards me and humiliates me yet again. I used to love Christmas, now I hate it. Happy times like birthdays and anniversaries and festive events are his favourite time to "relapse", as he calls it, and destroy our lives.

Walking back into the living room I hand him the can and smile stiffly, avoiding eye-contact. It's pointless as he's not looking at me anyway. "Ta, Baby", he mutters, taking the can from me as he leaves the room. I hear him go into the bedroom and shut the door again, and the urge to retch makes my eyes water.

"Dirty bastard", I mutter, and a tear forces itself out.

Sitting down on the chair near the window, I go online to see the likely victim he has on the go this time. Scrolling through his page, my eyes alight on a woman from his work. She occasionally sits on reception, looking like she's chewing a wasp. A mop of dark-rooted blonde curly hair, and lines that you could rest a pencil in all over her prematurely-aged face. Well, once he's done with her, she'll look like someone rolled her up and unravelled her, like a paper ball!

I know it's her. My sixth sense isn't what it used to be but every now and then the truth is like a bad smell. And I can smell whore and cheat all over this female, like the stench of a rotten, forgotten, bin!

At the Leisure Centre's Christmas night out a few days ago, she acted strange with me; following me to the toilet and wittering on at me about her "knowing Jamie better" than I did. I felt uneasy at the time and as usual my suspicion grew when, as she got more drunk, I caught her glaring at Jamie dancing with me or putting his hand on my knee.

Scowling at her profile picture, I look away to the mess in the living room. Gulping back shouts of rage and hurt, I try to drown them with what's left in my wine glass.

Yes, it's her. I don't feel the usual hurt, anger, or sickness; I actually feel sorry for her. Another colleague at the Leisure Centre, another mortified ex fuck-buddy. I close my phone and drop it to the floor and look outside. It's dark, but it's not snowing yet as the forecast said. In the glass, my sad face is reflected, and it makes me want to cry. As if watching a horror movie, I remember what it was like when we first met and had sex here, in this very living room, on that horrible red leather sofa.

Standing up, I wipe my hands on my bare legs as though wiping his sweat off me, and straighten the hem of my pyjama shorts. "Get a grip and get out Lola!" I whisper to myself as I start tidying the throws and fixing the cushions. Like it really matters now.

I never liked his flat anyway, moving in was a mistake. I wanted to live with him, thinking it would stop him cheating, drinking, and drugging. I think it's made him worse; now he knows I'm homeless if he discards me, or if I try to put a stop to his behaviour.

Thinking too deeply, looking out onto the frosty street as snow starts to fall, I've missed him creeping across the living room towards me. Turning to look at what's left to tidy before going to bed, I'm face to face with his crotch. Now he's undoing his belt. The sound of his denims dropping to the floor makes my throat tighten, but now I know this is the last time, I don't feel sick or afraid like he wants me to; I feel powerful.

Listen to: The Bee Gees – Jive Talkin'

Chapter 2: Running Water

Phoebe's next to me, wrapped in a blanket; she's usually made to sit on that blanket in the back. He's not here to insist where she can and can't sleep or sit anymore. This wonderful thought flies through me, hovers carefully then gently lands on the curve of my heart.

Turning the radio up, and flicking the heating on, I decide to accelerate out of the gravelled drive, loud enough to wake the dead. Well, the Devil himself perhaps! Looking in the rear-view mirror I see our bedroom light go on. It's 5am and the streets are deserted. Last night's snow has settled.

Phoebe barks in excitement; she's not used to us being out after dark. Her tongue lolling makes me want to smile, but I'm too nervous. I keep looking back to see if his car is behind me.

I've had nightmares about this moment for the last few weeks. Terrible dreams where he chases me and catches me and rapes me. Sharna looking on and laughing before he takes her hand. "Bye, fuckface!", I hiss under my breath as my phone starts buzzing in my pocket. "Your turn to be discarded and left to rot for once", saying this out loud helps my nerves; almost as though he could hear me.

****

Pretending to sleep as he dozed off, I'm laying in bed next to a sleeping Jamie. My eyes are scrunched up and closed so tight, I have a mild headache. Counting to 1000, each number carefully spaced apart, my heartbeat so loud I'm sure he'll hear it, and roll over to demand I stop breathing, so he can sleep better. He's back on the Valium, so I'm fairly confident I've just over 15 minutes to wait for him to be in a deep enough sleep so I can secure my exit from the bed.

The unusual sound of my sliding out from under the bedclothes and crawling across the floor wakes Phoebe, and she comes trotting in to see what she's missing. Ears pointing out aeroplane-style, she cocks her head and stops in the doorway, as I creep towards her.

Flicking her big brown eyes at the bed, it's as if she reads my mind. Frozen to the spot, praying she won't try and lick me or play at this, the worst moment she could choose, I shake my head at her roughly. My pony-tail catches my nose and I hold it tight; resisting the urge to sneeze. Blessedly, Phoebe turns and wanders away as if saying "Come on, then, mum. Let's get on with it".

On all fours, I drop my head in thanks, take another deep breath, and slowly stand up. Every part of my body tense and my face screwed up in comical concentration, as I try not to make even the slightest sound.

Avoiding the slightly-raised floorboard to the right of the door, I step one foot over, then the other; shoulders clenched and eyes shut, the fine hairs on the back of my neck stand to attention as Jamie mumbles something in the dark. I hold my breath until I hear the tell-tale creak of the bed as he pulls the bedcovers tighter around him.

I've packed only a small backpack for myself. I stuffed some extra things in my largest handbag and rammed some of Phoebe's food and a water bowl into a carrier bag just before bed, while he showered earlier. Tiptoeing along the dark gloomy hall, I'm waiting for him to yell for me from the bedroom. If he catches me creeping about at night, he will assume I'm checking his phone for filth and I will most likely receive a hit. If he's a little drunk and high on Valium that's actually more than likely; it's certain. My pyjama bottoms are too long and they whisper to me, as if encouraging me to hurry up, once I reach the kitchen.

Jamie likes me to sleep naked; "easy access" he's started to say recently. The escalation away from romance and love, and towards vile disrespect always speeds up when he cheats and takes drugs. The horror of knowing he was more sexually abusive towards me when he was feasting on other women, is a recent development. One that triggered a long-forgotten eating disorder last year.

Matching up his episodes of infidelity and excessive physical demands on me, made me sick for the first time in years. Food had become the enemy; after eating I was slower, less aware, and even though the women he was sexting and meeting were not exactly models, I felt so fat and ugly I wanted to disappear. Getting thinner and weaker, and choosing to either not eat or binge-then-purge, is one of the few things that I have control over now. Well, not for long! I'll make a better life somewhere else. I have to. Doing a "Sharna", and staying around to go in and out of his bed while stalking his abuse victims, is not on the cards for me; I'm damaged, angry, hurt and broken, but I have *some dignity intact*!

It would kill me. I might be a bitter and angry cow now, but that fate is far, far worse. "She used to be a nice person before she met him…", a friend from his AA group whispered to me the other day when I told her about Sharna's recent online comments about me. I looked at the friend in shock, and my plan to leave the pair of them to their evil escapades, to find myself again, became even more attractive.

Walking past the kitchen window, I catch sight of my reflection. I pause and stare back at the tiny, drawn person there. Big baggy pyjamas, even though they are a size 8. My short and thin ponytail, and the huge wide eyes of someone used to living with a full-blown anxiety disorder, are hard to miss. I don't want to be that person in the window anymore.

The self-loathing reached a new high, as the drinking to smother the constant anxiety replaced the food my body was lacking. Starving, not just for what used to be clean, kind love, but basic nutrients, had created a tremor in my right hand, my hair falling out and even my periods stopping. Yes, she's got to go. I leave her in the windowpane and set about the next part of my scary-as-Hell plan.

Going over and over how it's come to this, while attempting to retrieve a tracksuit, vest top, some fleece-lined boots, my biggest padded coat and a bobble hat from the washing machine has so far been the hardest part of this! The noise seems deafening in the dark, quiet house.

I thought getting it all in there was tough! Oh, how wrong I was! I sit back, take a breath and count to five before starting again. As the coat gives way with a gentle whoosh of the silky material, I let out a sigh of relief and Phoebe wanders into the kitchen. "Maybe wasn't the best idea, Pheebs" I whisper. She wags her tail then sits down to wait for me to finish this ridiculous mission.

Yes, frantic, I had to empty the washing machine of wet clothes and put my getaway gear in there instead! He never does any jobs like this, so the chances of him finding the clothes and suspecting my plan were zero.

As the shower stopped and I heard him flush the toilet, my heart jumped into my throat, so I slammed the door to the washing machine unusually hard. "What the fuck are you playing at?! Moody cow!" he yelled through the kitchen doorway as he stormed past and down the hall, naked and wet, heading for bed. "Sorry! I'll be in in a minute!" My voice desperately high and bright. "Just washing you some bits for the gym tomorrow!"

Dropping my pyjama bottoms to the floor and lifting the top over my head, I stand naked in the kitchen and smile grimly; this is the last time I'll be naked in here. Phoebe looks towards the hall quickly and cocks her head. My heart stops. If he walks in, I'll just pretend I was going to surprise him with sex over the kitchen table, again. My hands are shaking but I manage to dress quickly in the tracksuit, ram the hat on and clumsily put the coat on, wincing at how bloody noisy the material is!

****

Now, I'm nearly 50 miles away, heading south and, across long wide fields to my left, the sun's shyly appearing, setting fire to the blue-grey skies that threaten more snow.

Figuring early hours would be the best time to leave as the roads would be clearest, I chose before sunrise on Christmas Day and marked it in my online diary with a big red heart emoji, three days after Halloween. Knowing he usually slept most deeply before sun-up, this was a rare success.

Speeding along the almost empty motorway, I notice that away from the city there's a lot more snow. In most parts it's a good deal deeper than at home. Home? It's not my home anymore. Thank god.

Taking a sip of water from a bottle I found under the driver's seat, it's like I'm washing just a little of the dirt from the last few years off me. Talking aloud I give myself a bit of a pep talk. "Need to focus on moving forward. Focus on nice things: the scenery, where next, and a whole new year where I'll be safe".

Phoebe's been sound asleep for almost the entire journey but, on hearing my voice, she twitches a little and her ears perk up although she hasn't opened her eyes yet. Stroking her quickly then returning my hand to the wheel, my throat tightens in grief.

I don't think I would be here if it weren't for her. Here as in, *alive*... Jamie and Sharna have made me think about ending my own life several times, especially in recent months, since I left my job to "help him through another relapse". As usual, it was just him acting out under her pressure about child contact. He doesn't relapse, he just reacts! To her and any other challenge to his ego or his secret life. I really need to stop thinking about them. The whole point of leaving was to shed the rotten skin of their abuse.

Slowing a little and trying to centre myself by being mindful of my surroundings, I check to see if it's safe, and then pull over on the hard shoulder. Phoebe immediately wakes at the prospect of play, a walk, and a feed. I'm sorry to disappoint her. "Quick break, Pheebs, and then back in the car". I can actually feel her disappointment. She slows her trot towards the fence lining the fields around us, and puts her head down to sniff for a good place for a wee.

Stretching, and taking my hat off, I take in the view. It's icy cold but the sky is clear; it's going to be a nice day wherever we are headed. The snow's maybe a foot deep in some areas. It's frosted spindly trees into white-clothed skeletons, and cast diamonds over everything in sight. It's quite pretty, even for a motorway!

Starlings swoop and curl in the throbbing clouds above us. Phoebe comes to stand beside me, sits down but remains bolt upright, like a little lady. She's watching the birds intently and, like the snow, the rising sun has coloured her, everything but white. Bending down and ruffling her ears makes her turn to look at me, and I'm treated to The Staffy Smile.

"Now we just need to work out where the fuck we're going, Pheebs!" I try to laugh but my body isn't ready yet and tears threaten to come instead. Sensing my pain, she jumps up and tries lick me, and I have to push her back down to avoid muddy paw prints on my clothes.

Hearing a favourite song come on the radio, I encourage her back to the car and get in. Pulling out and back onto the road carefully, I turn the volume up a little and make myself sing along. Gently putting my foot down on the accelerator, I sing louder. South's good enough for now; anywhere far away from Jamie and Sharna will be perfect.

Listen to: Kiss – Lick It Up

Chapter 3: Bridgefell

My tummy started rumbling about a hundred miles ago. Not much of a surprise considering I haven't been able to bring myself to eat for the last four days. Not since I found that video of him masturbating, in a message stream to a woman on Facebook, yet again.

Of course, I didn't tell him I found it. The last time I confronted his cheating we were in bed; he kicked me so hard in the stomach, I flew several feet off the bed and across the room. My landing broke the television stand. Knowing better than to peel his mask away, at even the slightest hint he wasn't as perfect as he liked to appear to everyone else, was key. Every day was a school day with Jamie!

The hunger pangs are coming hard and fast now. I've lost a stone since I met him, and I was only eight stones in the first place! My tracksuit bottoms are a little loose, so I look ill. Checking my face in the rear-view mirror, I wince at how sick I look. My dark green eyes squint with tiredness and stress. I'm pale to the point of looking grey, and my lips are dry from dehydration. It's easy to underestimate how pain and betrayal can ruin your looks, until it happens to you.

I look like I have some kind of debilitating illness and I want to cry again. Poisoned from the inside out. His spit, cum, and lies inside me, rotting away at me, coring me out. "Oh! Shut up thinking, Lola!", I shout, and Phoebe sits up in fright. I need to change what I do to help me change how I think. "I need to eat; I need to find somewhere to stay, and replace what he took", I mutter.

Disgust sweeps over me, bringing with it the urge to retch. Then, a beautiful yellow and black sign; "service station with shower facilities, 10 miles" it reads. "Perfect!" I crow and Phoebe sits up to attention again. "Just like you…" I whisper, readjusting her collar so she's a little more comfortable. She Staffy-Smiles again.

Showering in a service station is a new thing for me; just like being single, in fact. Woah! I've not been single since I was a kid! The thought makes me feel a little ashamed. Am I that lost and needy that I've deliberately always had a bloke to lean on?

Scrubbing harder at my body, I'm punishing myself. Maybe that's how Jamie managed to keep me for so long. My own pathetic fear of being alone and adrift, with no one there for me.

With family scattered far and wide, parents and brothers all focused on their own lives, I've ended up too reliant on the wrong people. Never particularly good at female friendships, men became my family and my friends. One by one, I fell too hard, and too fast. And one by one, they disappointed me, or I disappointed them. Then Jamie came along. And my dreams, then my nightmares, came true.

I couldn't pack shampoo last night, so I'm using the soap dispenser on the wall of the cubicle. Smells ok but it's unusually foamy and promises dry, wildly knotted hair for the rest of the day. He won't like that; he hates my hair when it's messy. The thought happens like a promise I don't want to make. But, far away from him now, I let it sit there and simmer hot; a warning of how addicted I am to his abuse.

Stepping out of the cubicle, I realise I have to dry myself with paper towels. Sighing and regretting my terrible memory for details, like remembering to pack certain things, I finish dressing a few minutes later, just as a trucker walks in to freshen up.

"Oh, sorry!" he splutters and starts backing out in a panic. "It's ok, I'm finished now anyway. You go ahead". I don't make eye contact and I slide past him and outside quickly. That moment reminded me how cruel Jamie could be; I have had little to no privacy this last year. He started bursting in on me in the bath or shower, and a good few times while I sat on the toilet. He must have half a dozen pictures of me in my most vulnerable moments.

"Evil bastard", I mutter, walking across the car park. He's probably shared intimate pictures like that with his friends in AA. I caught him doing that with a few of the women he cheated on me with. Sharna will have been "shared about" too... "Gross", I spit and a woman walking past shoots me a look of surprise. I don't apologise. I feel angry all of a sudden. The waves of intense, negative emotion are unpredictable, but I'm used to it.

"Happy Christmas, honey", the silver-haired waitress says, as she slides purple spectacles to the top of her head, and offers a wide, red-lipped smile. Readying her pen above the order pad, she frowns a little as she realises I'm alone. Her bright blue eyeshadow catches the light and I want to ask her where she got it, but don't. I'm too chatty and I can't hide if I'm memorable or share too much.

"What's got you out and about on Christmas Day? It's freezing as well!". Embarrassed at my appearance, I tug the hood of my top over my head to hide my recently-washed hair. Looking up at her, I resist a blunt comeback along the lines of, This, so far, is the best Christmas Day I've had in a long time.

"Just travelling to my sister's, actually. Hubby's asleep in the car. Early start. Just wanted to grab a quick bite to eat before the last part of the journey". The lies come easily. Jamie's made sure I'm an excellent liar. I never was, before I met him.

"Well, the bacon's still fresh as it's only early still. Between you and me, it's not the best after nine! Mind you, neither am I. I start at four! The coffee's better than you'd think, too". She's kind, probably chats like this with all the customers. It's a small café, on a fast motorway, with a much bigger and busier service station only a few miles further on.

Over the last few months, maybe even as long as a year, I've developed a strange fear of busy places. He used to tense up if we walked into a busy supermarket or bar, get angry if I chatted to anyone, and particularly if he caught another man looking at me. Later, he'd punish me by ending the relationship, locking me out of the house, and then complete the cycle a day or so later with rough, extreme "make-up sex", as he called it.

"Well, I need something quick and easy to share with *him* outside. So… a bacon roll and one of your coffees then. Black. Strong. Wee bit of cold water in it, if that's ok?" My smile's wider now; I've just realised I don't need to listen to his accusations of my attention seeking or "deliberate flirting" anymore. I can go where I like, look at who I like, and speak to who I like!

"Sure - five minutes and I'll be right back". She starts to walk away, then turns. "Lovely accent! Where in Scotland are you from?" My gut drops; this means she'll remember me. If he decides to come looking, or simply calls the string of service stations along the motorway, this woman will remember me. The tiny, wet-haired young woman with a Scottish accent, in a distinctive green Mini. Sitting all alone at 8am on Christmas Day, pretty much in the middle of nowhere. The Hubby thing won't deter her. It's not enough.

Thoughts racing, I try to come up with something to put her off. Another red herring. Any red herring! Shit! I can't have him find me. I don't mean in the physical sense, but online. If he knows where I end up, he can search there for me using social media, company website staff lists and even any groups or clubs I might join.

One of his exes warned me, this is what he does. He stalks anyone who gets away from him and makes their lives as miserable as he can. Livid that he lost control.

Going by Sharna's behaviour towards me, I have an instinct she will stalk and harass me wherever I go, too. Again, using social media. Why she's so obsessed with who her ex dates is beyond me. It's not as if Jamie's a catch!

"Oh! No, no, no! I'm not Scottish! It's a habit I picked up at work, saying *"Wee"*. I'm as Northern as they come. Lancaster!" Thank god my parents were Northern, although I was born in Scotland! Mind you, I've always been good at accents.

"Oh! We used to holiday in Scotland when I was a lass! That's going back years ago now. In fact, so long ago that the dinosaurs were still lumbering about!" She cackles and throws her head back at her own joke. The thought makes me want to laugh, but I've slipped up. I need to leave as quick as possible. I look at my watch and smile at her and say nothing. It's uncomfortable. I hate being rude.

She frowns again, but doesn't ask anymore and heads towards the kitchen. I think I see her falter as though she wants to come back and chat more, but she seems to change her mind and disappears behind the counter. Thank goodness for that! That little scare's taken the edge off my appetite but not enough to have me bolting for the door empty-handed. It does smell really good in here.

A few minutes later I've torn the roll in two and, holding one half in my mouth, I reverse out of the small car park and put my foot down to carry on southbound. Phoebe munched her half in two bites so, realising I'm not sharing my half, let out a small grunt then settled down to sleep again. I've decided where to go. Cornwall. They'll never find me there, not a snowball's chance in Hell.

The canteen lady was right, the coffee was spectacularly good. The lift of caffeine and full belly has kept me going for a few more hours. Phoebe asleep next to me, occasionally twitching or whining, chasing dream bunnies or, more likely, boy dogs, makes me smile more than once.

Wherever we go, she will be happier too. He was never cruel to her, just not interested in her. Too focused on his own needs. It was her adoration of me that got on his nerves and made me extra anxious which, in turn, made her unsettled and needy.

Thank god I don't have any children! Imagine putting them through three years of our dramas, my tears and his unpredictability and, worst of all, his lack of care for anyone but himself! Now the cycle's broken, and it's just going to be us. A ripple of relief drifts over me but dissipates fast. True, I might have a destination in mind, but no further plans beyond that. Typically impulsive, but not typically a risk taker, this situation has me anxious again.

As the miles slip under the wheels of the car, I get closer to Cornwall and the pressure mounts. How the hell am I going to make this work? Leaving him was surprisingly easy, but staying away from the cycle of adoration then abuse wasn't easy before. This is the first proper "ending", but not the first time I've been forced out of our relationship.

He must have dumped, or "discarded", me (as it's called in these types of relationships) a hundred times or more. It's created a sense of addictive, self-harming behaviours where I've begged to be let back in, even though I know once inside his house and his bed, I'm right back where I started: under his control and vulnerable to whatever horrible thing I'm going to discover, or whatever disgusting message stream he's involved in, *yet again*.

Few people could understand it. Our so-called friends watched the fallout then make-up, over and over again and often questioned my patience, as well as Sharna's obsession. I rarely had answers for them and, when I did, it broke me and has brought me here. Once I'm in Cornwall, I'm going to bury all this deep inside and make a new life. I'm going to totally ignore the memories and thoughts, and hide the emotions so well I can't find them again.

"Once I get to Cornwall, it's done! Gone! All of it!". Another car passes me and the driver catches me talking to myself. Well, shouting really. I cringe in embarrassment and look away.

"Cornwall, 16 Miles", the sign slides past. It's nearly 10am and, bizarrely, I want to cry. The last time I was here, I was 15. Just over 20 years ago now. A school trip. Two weeks at a campsite in the hottest May for decades. Going through my plain, mousy, and slightly dumpy stage, I was bullied for my accent and called "Man" at the time.

I think it was nearly a year before any of the other children referred to me by my actual name. Perhaps it was this depersonalisation of me - the brutal inhumane way that I wasn't my own gender, simply because I had short hair - that pushed me even further down the path of choosing the company of boys, and then men.

I would sit alone in the toilets at break times to avoid the catcalls, the finger-pointing and "Hi, Man", "Where you going, Man?", "What's for lunch, Man?", harassment and cackling, mostly by girls but, of course, some boys too. Later, those boys would be the ones chasing me. Making the girls bitter that "Man" had bloomed into someone prettier and slimmer than they were.

Once I grew breasts, started showing off the long legs my parents insisted I hide in thick tights and old-fashioned knee-length corduroy skirts, I swiftly learned that the way to protect myself from the bullying was to make sure the boys wanted me, more than the girls bullied me. That was the beginning of the end of who I could have been. My neediness, low self-esteem, and fear of being on my own, has made me vulnerable to being used by men. I've traded sex for what I perceived as acceptance and respect.

I'd forgotten all about that school trip until, walking out of the café and passing the maps and postcard stand, my eye caught a small row of seashells. Each shell had "I like to be beside the seaside" handwritten on them. Not specifying a place alongside the writing, they likely didn't mean Cornwall in particular. But something about their pale pink, blue and yellow, triggered the bittersweet memories.

Walking alone on the beach, before we were called to breakfast, enjoying the peace and quiet, I wandered the shore and collected shells every day of that trip. Always one to enjoy the outdoors, especially anywhere near the sea, I must have cast a slightly sad figure all on my own, not a friend in sight and up so early while my classmates typically slept as late as was feasibly possible. I don't think it's normal for someone not quite 16 to be collecting shells, I really was quite naïve and immature as a teenager. Until well, let's not go there just now.

A lump in my throat, I turn the music up again and open the window for fresh air. I don't want to think about all that stuff. I'm best on my own now. No one's coming near me or my body again.

Now I'm angry. That's better. Anger is better. Being sad always sent me back to him. It's time I get angry and get better. Whatever "better" means!

The sun's higher now – well, as high as it gets in the dead of Winter. As we get further south, the land's lusher. The snow has melted here to reveal pretty, winding, roads with the promise of the sea, just slightly twinkling in the distance. I really need a drink.

The thought slaps me in the face, and the shame of how low I've sunk in the name of love, makes me breathless. I'll get that sorted too. I can't believe I've ended up like him. The sexual things, the alcohol and even drugs, once! All to try and appease him, calm myself or even make sense of what was going on in his head. Desperation isn't the word for it. I don't know what is.

****

"Cheer me up baby...." Jamie whines, as he puts my hands on his crotch. My palms and sleeves are still wet from wiping tears away for the last three hours. Begging him to please tell

me why he keeps doing what he does. Begging him to stop Sharna from making us miserable. "You're imagining it. It's not real. You're paranoid. Now, cheer me up so we can make up properly". He pushes my dress up...

* * * * * * * * * * * * *

The flashback crashes in so fast and hard, I swerve a little onto the grass verge. It gives me such a fright, I press the brakes hard. Phoebe clings to the seat with her claws to stop herself falling into the footwell. She looks at me in such shock that I do start to cry then. Car half on, half off the verge on the quiet, tree-lined road. Cows peering over the dry-stone wall next to me, I sob and sob until my chest hurts.

The low hum of an approaching car coming up the hill towards me shakes me awake. I'd fallen asleep at the wheel with Phoebe on my lap. "Fuck!" The last thing I need is anyone asking awkward questions or noting my presence here. I'm sticking out like a sore thumb as it is.

I duck down in the seat as the car slows down and passes. I can feel the driver trying to see inside my car, but I'm so small I've managed to get into the footwell.

Only once the car has passed do I uncurl myself. The need for a drink flutters in my chest again, but this time the shame doesn't. "Anyone going through what I have would be a raging alcoholic, as it is!" Muttering to myself, I carefully pulling the car off the verge and ease onto the road.

Phoebe makes her little gremlin sound, telling me she's thirsty and hungry. This confirms my plan to stop soon. "Yep, we'll stop at the next village and have a think, sweetheart". Her tail flickers but she doesn't Staffy-Smile at me; she really is ready for a comfort break.

"Bye Bye, nosey cows", I call out of the window and start to drive down the road. One of the animals has the cheek to moo at me and swish her tail, I see the tip of it above the wall. The comedy of it cheers me up a little. Being far away from what used to be home, and heading towards the coast, already has me feeling lighter and fresher. I'm sure coming south and settling here will have me better in no time at all.

I open Phoebe's window and watch as she sits to attention in excitement. A waft of cow manure reminds me of home, of the island where I was raised. Funny how, there, I apparently had an English accent and down here it's Scottish. That reminds me, I need to watch how I talk. Small places have loud voices. And gossip will be my biggest enemy if I want to be anonymous.

The scenery out here really is beautiful. Rolling green fields pocked with mini forests; giant hedges beautifully-shaped and almost smooth, as though sculpted by a giant. Driving under long tunnels of trees, where the sunlight dapples the damp but thawing frosty road, is mesmerising.

It's all downhill now, and there's a scent of the sea on the breeze. Phoebe's nose is twitching, and she has her paws on the dashboard while her tail wags hard. But I know she will be thirsty, so stopping soon is really important. The roads are narrow and occasionally a small farmhouse or cottage watches us drive past.

There's a little wooden hand-painted sign ahead, I guess correctly that it's for the name of whatever village or town is about to greet us. Slowing and stretching to peer out of the window, I stop and read aloud; "*Bridgefell. Honestly, the best village in Cornwall!*" I chuckle at the over-confident sign and wonder who made it. "Says here, it's only another two miles 'til this Bridgefell. That's good!" Putting the car in gear again, and setting off slowly, I chat to Phoebe excitedly.

"Right. If it has a beach or even some rocky shoreline, we are definitely stopping, Pheebs. You can have a drink and a walk around and I can have a drink and well, a walk around!" She turns and gets up to look out of the window again. My heart lifts: things will be fine. It's all going to be fine.

A few minutes later, the village comes into view. It's tiny! So small I can see the sea and I'm barely in the centre yet! Cruising past whitewashed cottages and idyllic gardens, plush and filled with colour even though it's December, I notice that the village has a rather unique shape. Split in two, it seems to have an upper and a lower part. I like it. "Quaint and quirky! I'm liking it here already!" I mutter. "Maybe I won't carry on along the coast. You never know, this might be worth a longer visit..." Phoebe's tail wags harder and she lets out a couple of "Yips" in excitement.

At the bottom of the hill, I can see the sea glistening as though it's high summer. Then into view comes a small, pebbled beach, a little pier and even, to finish the picture, a cluster of bobbing boats. "This'll definitely do!" We pull into a small car park beside a pub. The sign above the door, black with gold writing, is fresh-paint pristine, and reads "The Pint and Pebbles".

"If I had a pub, I'd call it The Gin and Lobster" I say for probably the hundredth time to no one in particular, as Phoebe and I walk towards the entrance. Pushing the door open with Phoebe close on my heels, I narrow my eyes to the darkness inside. It's not yet lunchtime so it's not surprising to see it deserted – although I am surprised the door's unlocked and the bar itself has no one serving, or at least watching the till.

Feeling a bit awkward, I think we should perhaps have that walk first then come back in a bit. As I start to open the door to head back outside, a voice calls. "Hi! Are you in for some lunch?" The bar's quite dark and it takes me a few seconds to see a woman in a booth in the furthest corner. I'd missed her, her dark hair against the deep red of the leather seating, and the shadows, rendered her virtually invisible.

"More a drink really. Long drive. Can my pup come in too? Like, is it dog-friendly?" I'm walking towards her and can see her more clearly now. She's older than me, could be described as attractive, but looks shorter than me and a little plumper.

I hold my hand out and smile a hello, but it's ignored as she stands up and walks away from me and behind the bar, calling over her shoulder, "What would you like?" She disappears from view before I can answer, but reappears with a silver dog bowl filled with water. Phoebe's standing up with her front paws flat on the sides of the bar and panting in excitement. New people, a pub and fresh water - pretty much her favourite three things all in one.

"I'll have a pint of lager with some lime cordial in, please". I take the bowl and place it in the corner by the booth where the woman had been sitting, and Phoebe pushes past me to get to it and attacks the water voraciously.

"Must have been a long drive! She's thirsty as hell!" the woman laughs. She's expecting me to say where I came from.

"A bit. I was on my way to make a surprise visit to my sister further down the coast, but when I called her, she's only flipping gone abroad this year! My fault, not hers. Typical me - cock up and on Christmas Day as well."

"Well, we're quiet now, but every year we have a village Christmas dinner and party in here. I try and stay open all year round. You're welcome to join in. It's a small enough place for us to do that. One of the perks of being in the middle of nowhere, and there aren't many!" She's pouring the pint and my mouth waters at the thought of it. If we stay here tonight, then I can have more than one. A lot more than one...

"How cool! Only problem is, I've nowhere to stay..." Phoebe stops drinking and looks at me. Water drips from her jaw onto the stone floor. The woman hands me a paper towel and I bend to wipe Phoebe's dribble.

"I let rooms out. Only three of them. I have the flat on the top floor. I keep the guest areas simple, but clean and cheap. *Like me!*" she says and lets out such a loud guffaw I jump. "Woah, you're skittish!" she says and frowns, but softens it with a smile.

"I've always been a bit... on edge. Don't take offence. Being tired always makes it worse".

"None taken", she says, throwing the used paper towel in the bin below the bar. I take a long pull on the lager as she turns her back to fetch a key from a row of hooks further down the bar. "Have a think about it. It's only fifty a night, no breakfast, but you're not an eater, I can tell!"

Flushed with embarrassment, I look down at my clothes and how badly they hang off me, especially now crumpled from the last seven hours' driving. "I've not been well recently". Smoothing the top down across my chest and pulling the waistband up a little, I hope I look slightly less urchin-like.

"Well, you've come to the right place to recuperate. Sea air, sandy blokes, and a pub. What more could you want?! Just ask Carolanne and she will sort you out!" Carolanne's handing me the key and a pen for the guest ledger.

"Why not? Best offer I'm going to get today. Aaaaand Phoebe likes it here". Smiling, I glance over to where she's sat down: on Carolanne's magazine, on the seat of the booth where she'd been sitting.

"My name is...". I search for a fake name, but give up as the time stretches between us and Carolanne watches me closely. "Lola...", I sigh in resignation; I don't want to lie any more than I need to. I hate lying, but it's been a necessity this last while to try and cope with always having to appease and avoid Jamie's mood swings and Sharna's constant stalking.

The room's small but warm. There's a view over the rear of the pub, onto their storage area, but it's not a big deal. And, if I lean out of the window far enough, I can just see the edge of the beach and smell the sea.

Slightly tipsy from the two pints downstairs, I wander around the room and nosey in cupboards and check out the bathroom. I'm pleased it's got a bath and not just a shower. That way I can try my usual way of relaxing: a long hot bath and a drink. "I can wash my wetsuit in here too. That's good...".

I usually leave my swimming gear in the back of the car, ready for whenever I need it. Jamie used to complain that the wetsuit in particular took up too much space in the wardrobe. Considering he only ever hung his clothes up on the floor or rammed them into drawers, I was surprised he even knew I had a wetsuit in the wardrobe! "Wanker", I mutter, roughly pulling clothes out of my bag.

I've packed three swimming costumes, as well as my sea-swimming kit. I plan on getting my times up and building fitness again. In the first two years of our relationship, I was super-fit. But once he became his true self, and the toxicity started to affect me, I stopped swimming and going to the gym; I knew everyone he worked with and likely worked out with, knew what he had been doing there. The women. The sex. And worst of all, me being one of them. It all put me off going to the Leisure Centre, and I became the most isolated and shy I have ever been in my life. And coming from someone maladjusted as I am, that's really saying something!

The memory of when we first met, at the pool in the centre where he worked, hits me full force between the eyes. In my hand is the red "Baywatch" swimming costume I bought when he was chasing me. A whole six months before we became intimate. *That girl*, the one who would wear *this*, needs to come back. I need her to.

"I'm going to be me again! Fuck him!" Phoebe looks up in mild alarm at yet another one of my outbursts. The urge to sit on the floor and call Jamie... is *suffocating*.

Here we go. The intrusive thoughts have started. They usually consist of denial, regret, shame, and panic. It's the same every time I try to leave him.

Sitting heavily on the bed, the familiar feelings of early detox from Jamie have my temperature dropping and fingers itching to reach for the phone. It's like a tape on rewind. Hurtling backwards, I'm skipping the bad bits and pausing on the good bits.

The romantic songs he'd sing, the sex in the early days when it was equal and satisfying, tender even. The long hot baths together and short cold days walking through our hometown. *Could he change?* Maybe he's already booking himself back into rehab? Put Sharna back in her place as long-term ex and just a plain old baby-mama to him. I bet he's started blaming her for me running away from him.

To be honest, she's worse than he is. He has his mental issues and sex addiction problems, and drugs and booze, and bad upbringing to blame... she's an *ex one-night stand!* Stalking me and harassing him... that makes no sense. None at all... Yes, the denial and fear of being without him is in full torrential flow now. Right on time. I glance at my phone and my fingers tingle with the desire to call Jamie.

"If I unpack, I'm less likely to run to the car and head straight home", I mutter to myself. Folding clothes neatly and putting them in drawers and hanging them in the wardrobe, I force myself to settle in and think about the here and now. *Not him and her.*

As I take out the half a dozen items I packed, my nerves start to fray; I'm really nervous about this Christmas party thing. A room packed with complete strangers and so many questions is going to be a tough one to navigate. What was I doing leaving him? Coming here? This was a horrendous idea! Maybe this time he will change? Be better? Go back to NA and work more honestly in AA?

He's been calling and texting all day and I've managed to successfully focus on the journey and not reply or listen to any of the voicemails. I'll do that later, when I'm brave enough. Waiting until tomorrow would be better, a record for me!

Maybe I could just check online? On his pages? See if he's trying to reach out to me there? He's done it before, he's sure to do it again. He uses our friends as middlemen to show off how much he loves me when we are together. On a few occasions he's used them to get messages to me, when he hasn't had the guts to do it himself. He likes talking to me when I'm blocked on one site, by using another. It's a clever way of showing people he's moved on when he hasn't. I am often his dirty secret, although we are in a long-term relationship. I hate it! No, *I hated it*! Past tense.

"Stick with the plan, Lola!" I tell myself, while pouring a gin from the small half bottle I packed last night, and the ice bobbing in the fizz, the familiarity of it, has me back at home, in the living room. Waiting for him to come in from work so I can surprise him with a favourite dinner or sexy outfit.

Ok - it's just one look. One quick scroll to see how upset he is. It doesn't mean I'm going back but it will make me feel a bit better. If he's upset, he will be more likely to consider going clean and sober again, maybe even finally getting a court order to see his baby with Sharna. "She's the problem. The knife in my back. The thorn in my side. I can fix him. But her? She's way past saving!"

I'm tapping the screen to enter my password without even considering how dangerous and stupid this is. My phone's gone flat on the long drive. Fate saves me from contacting him, and I plug the phone in, with a weak sense of gratitude. I was always so controlled and sensible before I met him. Well, not entirely. But a lot more than I am now.

I can hear the sound of people through the floorboards. It's mid-afternoon and the party's starting. God, I wish he were here. I wish he never turned so dark. I wish she never started on us or even existed, in fact! I wish I were better on my own. Wish, wish, fucking wish!

Drinking back what's left in the glass, I snatch at my phone as soon as it hits 2% and allows me to turn it on. Within a minute I'm logging into Facebook and start to scroll down the feed. After 20 minutes, I still can't see anything of note. Having had another two drinks in the search time, I start to see double and get a little bored.

I don't really know what the lack of posts on his page means. Usually he's online posting over and over how much he loves me. Or he's simply invisible, having blocked me. No in-betweens, no... nothing, like this. I can see his profile and hers, and neither have posted anything yet today. Sharna likes to gloat when he and I have our mini-splits, even though it's not exactly beneficial to her. They've not been an item for a few years. Not to mention that Jamie always insisted it was the odd one-night stand, almost always manufactured by her.

Regularly blocking and unblocking me, she's predictable. Me being unblocked means she has something to brag about, probably another new bloke. She'll end up with four kids by four blokes soon enough... He's probably sleeping off his hangover and will get started on social media once he feels less like dying. I'm not there to cook him a meal, or bring glass after glass of water while he lies in bed on his phone, watching porn on XHamster, or sexting strangers and customers from his workplace.

There! Now, that spurt of anger has helped a bit! Maybe the flashbacks and memories aren't so pointless after all. "Bath-time! Pheebs!" She puts her head down and her ears back in dread. "Not you. Not this time!" I laugh, as I make another drink and eye up the bathroom.

The music downstairs is a bit louder now. The smell of food has turned musky and sour. The dinners have been eaten and the drinking's in full flow. Stomachs lined. The whole pub is enjoying Christmas Day and I'm here, alone and almost drunk, like a total loser. I'm just drunk enough to not cry in self-pity and consider what I might wear tonight, if I dare go downstairs.

Stripping off, casting clothes lazily in a path from the bed to the bathroom, I stumble a little on the recently-cleaned floor. Carolanne has used a bit too much detergent and the floor's slippery. I can check his page again later. He's texted and called all day, so the online silence is weird but not the only example of how sorry he is - yet again.

Sinking into the water, I close my eyes in shame. My previously slightly-rounded belly is long gone, and my hips stick up like icebergs from the steaming water. I want to cry again. Why would anyone want to hurt another human being, like he's hurt me? I don't understand it. He had all the sex and intimacy he, or any man, could ever want. After that first time, I never once said no.

Running my hands over my thighs and down my calves, I let a sob escape. He was so loving in the beginning. Passionate yes, determined certainly, but never ever did I think he'd turn so... oh, I don't know! It's all fair and well one of his exes telling me about NPD, but it's all too much! Understanding some of why he has been so abusive and manipulative has helped a tiny amount. But years of handling all those lies, the images in my head, his changeable-like-the-weather moods and her, oh god her! She's been *relentless*.

I feel a bit sick. Maybe I should eat something. Phoebe's going to be hungry again. When is she ever not hungry?! Almost as if reading my mind, she pads into the bathroom and sits on the bathmat, cocking her head at me in her usual "Come on, then. What's next?" way.

"Make me a drink and we can talk" I say firmly. She Staffy-Smiles at me and I smile back, then dip my head under the water to rinse the last of the conditioner away. Under the water, in my own favourite place, a buzzing sound gets through to me. My phone! It's him. He's going to say he's checked into rehab! Maybe this time, he's had such a scare, we can go back to where we were!

Rearing up out of the water, I splash Phoebe and the floor so much that she runs from the bathroom, tail between her legs. The bed squeaks as she leaps up on to it, away from the possibility of getting wet again.

"Sorry, Pheebs!" I call, virtually leaping out of the bath. I'm a bit dizzy. The lack of food with drink hasn't been helped by a far too hot bath. The phone's still buzzing, but it's not Jamie. It's a dog-walker I know. "Why's she calling me?" My heart squeezes and then I remember Phoebe's with me, not her - it's not about her. "Fucksakes, get it together, Lola".

"Hi, Pen! Whashup?!" The words smudge together with the alcohol, and I feel a pang of shame. "I'm away with a friend at the moment". I lie so easily these days. Pretending to have friends. Pretending he's ok. Pretending I'm ok. Pretending I still know who I am.

"Haven't you seen?...", my friend pauses and seems to be collecting different words from the ones she was going to say. Maybe there's been another dog stolen from our local supermarket or that dodgy dog-walker guy finally done for not picking shit up.

"Spit it out, Pen! Seen what?"

"He's with her. Your guy. He's *with* her, *with her*. With that mad ex, the Sharna One. The one you said was causing problems. He's back *with her*. She started posting all these videos and pics on her Facebook pages about 10 minutes ago. The internet is broken, Lola! Jeez! What the fuck is that about?!".

Dropping the phone on the floor, I fall to my knees and howl.

****

Someone's calling my name. There's knocking, too. Pen's voice stopped a while ago. She hung up when I didn't reply. Maybe my crying freaked her out. The water on the floor's cooled and I'm still naked. Disorientated, I'm trying to work out what the knocking sound is.

"Lola?! Are you ok? I heard....noises...sounded like crying? From your room? Is the dog ok? I forget her name now. Can you let me in?" It's Carolanne. The woman from the pub. The pub I'm staying in, now. Shit. *Omg - he's with her?!* Sharna and him? Our stalker and him?! They're together? Fucking? *Having sex?*

Crawling to the toilet, I retch loudly and Carolanne knocks harder. I don't want to see her, or anyone, ever again. The clickety clack of Phoebe's claws on the floor behind me signals her coming to investigate. She starts to whine; that same whine she uses when I used to cry when he cheated on me or locked us out of the house. It's high pitched, over and over like a baby getting ready to go full-on wail.

Babies, we never had any. It was a dream for me at first to have a child with him, then it became a nightmare. Sharna scrabbled at getting pregnant on purpose to create a permanent excuse. A Link. A Tie. Binding her forever with Jamie. He said this, and I came to agree with him. For once, he told the truth. "Had that kid on purpose to trap me!" was his mantra at the end of the month, as I paid the maintenance for him or paid another bill so *he could pay it.*

"Lola, I have a spare key. I'm coming in. I need to make sure you're ok. I'm counting to five then opening the door whether you like it or not" She sounds cross rather than worried now, and I feel bad for her.

How many times have I humiliated myself in front of complete strangers? Snot, tears, and pain-stained clothes all showing me up as I sat in bars, parks, or the stairwell at his flat. Constantly sobbing over him, his lies, and his filth. Now it's going to be *their filth*. Again. Fresh agony rips through my gut and I bend over in pain to silent-howl again.

I can't have her walking in and seeing me this bad. I need to try and get myself together, even a bit. "Wait a second. I'm coming". Blowing my nose on the edge of a towel, I smooth my wet hair back and wrap the towel around me. Slowly, stepping over the wettest parts of the floor, I wince as I see how wet the carpet into the bedroom is now. Phoebe's sat by the door, shaking slightly; ridges up, ears back. "I'm sorry, baby" I whisper and gently nudge her out of the way and open the door.

"Jesus hell! What the fuck happened to you! She's red with alcohol and a bit sweaty. I'm not surprised. The smell of Christmas Dinner and other people's perfumes and aftershaves assaults me as she pushes hard and the door opens fully. "Let's get you sorted and take you down for a drink. You need out of this room! I've not missed that you've been up here all afternoon and its nearly seven!"

She begins to step past me then stops as someone shouts for her, a little further down the hall and out of sight. "Mum! Folk are asking where you are?!" His voice gets louder towards the end of the hall and then a face appears. The young man blushes when he sees I'm only in a towel and quickly steps back from sight.

"Sorry. Ummmm, Mum, you need to come. Someone said you'd do the raffle. Riley's too pissed to do it and Mrs Borland's bought six tickets and wants to go home". He laughs and for some reason I smile. It's a deep laugh and I can imagine some old lady stood with her tickets all fanned out, expecting a win, and refusing to go home until she gets one.

"Let me sort Lola out, then come down. Whatserface can wait for five minutes. Get her a double sherry on the house, and tell her she can have an extra ticket. Seven is her lucky number. There! Crisis averted". Carolanne winks at me and steps inside the room. I hear her son walk down the corridor and jog down the stairs. I'm surprised he seems so compliant.

"Let's have a look for something for you to wear, Miss Cry Baby!" Yep, I think it's the drink and the heat that has her a bit short-tempered. She's very different to how she was downstairs, that's a fact. "What do you have in the wardrobe?" She's already opening the doors and flicking through the meagre set of clothing I brought. A low-cut white linen shirt, my wetsuit, my coat, a scarf, a couple of vest tops and my favourite red cotton skirt.

"Not this, too tarty" she says, throwing the skirt out of the wardrobe. "This is fine!" She casts the shirt at me, and it hits my face. I feel a prick of annoyance. She is drunk. Yep! She is one of *those* today: an annoying and rude drunk. I'm glad that's not my style, no matter how much booze I throw down my neck.

"Jeans? Trousers? Where are they?" She's searching the drawers now and happily throws my only pair of denims at me. "That's you sorted. A shirt and jeans". `

To be honest, it's what I would have worn anyway. The skirt is for when I don't mind being noticed; once I'm back to my old self. "I have trainers or heels, Carolanne. Don't dare say the trainers, either!". She frowns at my mild cheek then hands me the heels that I had on the shelf of the wardrobe. I'd put them away out of sight. The red PVC stilettos remind me too much of happier times with Jamie; I love these shoes but not how they make me feel. Mind you, by wearing them tonight I'm cancelling out all the times that they sat on my feet as I sat alone, crying, and waiting for him to end a discard and let me back into his favour.

"Sure, heels it is, moody cow!" She throws them on the bed, and I wince. This makes my head pound even more. Any facial movement, actually, hurts right now! I've been having migraines in response to stress for the last few months. The surges in cortisol and adrenalin up and down, over and over again, have put my body out of sync; I can't help but react in an extreme way, even in mildly stressful situations. Carolanne makes me nervous and I don't know why.

Putting my head in my hands and closing my eyes, hoping for relief from the pain, I realise there's a scent of stomach acid from where I forgot to flush. As if reading my mind, she interrupts the fresh thoughts of going home with another set of demands. "You clean your teeth, get dressed and move yourself downstairs ASAP. Carolanne is NOT taking no for an answer". She points at herself with her thumb and sways a little and I offer a half-smile even as my chest tightens in mild fear. Bossy people trigger me. Controlling people really trigger me!

"Ok. I won't take long. My hair's nearly dry anyway and I deffo do need a drink". I don't have the energy to argue with her, even if I wanted to. I put my feet in the denims and stop to look up at her. "Can you get me some painkillers, do you think?" She's watching me pull my denims up; even at a size

24-inch waist, they're a bit big for me. Too late to be shy now; I'm halfway to plastered and all the way to embarrassed.

"No problem. I'll get you downstairs in a few minutes and, if you don't hurry up, I'm sending up reinforcements". She's gone before I can say anything else.

Listen to: *Del Amitri – Always The Last To Know*

Chapter 4: Dirty, Dirty Men!

I know I shouldn't have looked. I should have just simply ignored it. Normal people don't go looking for pain. Normal people just get on with things. Get on with their lives by licking wounds. Deflecting the sticks and stones. Getting over one man by getting under another. Yep, normal people are supposed to do all that crap.

But all that shit is reserved for normal people. *I'm not normal.* I've not been normal in a long time. How can I be normal when Jamie wasn't? When Sharna wasn't? When what I had to do, to be allowed to sleep, or eat or work, or not be discarded from his life *wasn't*?

My phone feels hot in my hand, although I'm cold all over. The video of Jamie and Sharna in the park is on loop. I'm replaying each time it finishes. Over and over I watch them push their child on the swings. I hear it giggle and squeal. At exactly the same spot, I flinch at Sharna's big loud, proud, and spiteful laugh. Time and time again, I close my eyes at his false, overly excited one, fuelled by spite and Valium. Both glorying in their win. Both knowing I'd see this bizarre charade and want to die. Just like I do now.

There's such a sickness in them loathing each other, blaming the innocents lured into their game, then falling "madly" in love again. And doing it all over social media. I hate him. I hate her. I have no plans to go back to him and be all buddy-buddy or have sex, knowing that infidelity and rage are the very foundations of what they feed off. Why - no - *how* do they have the ability to do that?!

Ah! This explains his silence online. But, of course, she won't know he's called and texted all day, or made me suck the life out of him last night, before he happily got in the shower - again. Yeah, that late night shower was probably an opportunity to message her or call her, with the sound of running water covering up his tapping and masturbation.

She won't know that *I'm* the one who ended it, and ran like a rat from an already-sunken ship. There's something rancid and rotten about what's happening here. It's taking my every last ounce of energy not to scream and scream and pull every hair out of my head. The only reason I'm not is because of Carolanne. She's already made it clear she can hear my wails, and it's been a good 15 minutes since she told me to get ready and join her and all these happy, lucky, strangers downstairs.

I've brought some of his Valium with me. Stupid, I know, but worthwhile. Because right now, I think it might just stop me overdosing on the anti-depressants I've hoarded, since I realised they didn't suit me, several months ago. In the full-length mirror by the bed, I look thinner and more ghostly than before. It's like someone drew in the bathroom steam to let my outline drip downwards, like I'm actually melting away to nothing, just a small puddle of tears on the bedroom floor...

Decision made, I take two of the Valium and another quick drink. That's the bottle finished now, so avoiding downstairs is not an option anymore if I want another drink.

I finish dressing slowly. Within five minutes, a warm, fuzzy feeling starts from behind my ears, and spreads down my chest, arms, belly and, lastly, takes root in my toes. The only way to describe it, is the sun just came up, but inside my head, inside my head, chasing the shadows away, shining a light on the why. *This. This is why he did it?* This is why Diazepam is Jamie's drug of choice. Interesting. Wow! Yes, it really works!

Tossing the phone into my clutch bag, I start to button the white shirt I'd already chosen before... before... och! Who cares?! Those fuckers are welcome to each other. It's only a matter of time until he crucifies Sharna and dumps his kid again, readying himself to lure in another innocent to be their plaything and target of choice. Good! Let someone else be in agony for a change.

There's a small radio in the corner, by the tea and coffee stand, so I turn it on. Already tuned into a popular music channel, my need for music is well-timed. A song he once sent me fills the small room and my stomach turns to stone but my brain, for once, doesn't join in. These things are good!

"Highly addictive and best avoided at all costs" His GP had said last time I dragged Jamie to the surgery, to beg for help with his addictions. "It's the drugs that make me do it" was, and probably still is, his favourite excuse for the abuse.

Do I care right now? Nah. In fact, I don't really care about anything. Nothing and no one in this world gives a damn about me, and no more will I give a damn about them. Nope, nada, zilch. Not gonna happen. "It's dog eat dog now, Pheebs", I slur at her perfectly round, curled-up shape under the duvet. Beneath it, her tail flickers into life, and she wags it, making me laugh. It's a strange laugh: metallic, higher than usual, and staccato like a gun.

"Excuse me? I've been told to come and get you?" The voice is muffled behind the door, but I know who it is. It's Carolanne's son.

"Just one minute, putting a face on and promise I'm coming down!" I hope he doesn't wait for me.

"Mum says I'm to wait for you. No arguments", he replies.

"Fuck", I hiss. Frantically putting on my usual minimal make-up, and making as good a job as I can while a bit high and more than a bit drunk, the warpaint takes exactly a minute, and I'm strangely pleased with myself. These pills aren't just happy pills, they make you actually *like* yourself! "He really was onto something wasn't he? My Jamie". I whisper, opening the blankets and stroking Phoebe a gentle goodbye. She opens one eye, half-heartedly wags her tail, then loudly snuffles her nose deeper into the curve of her belly.

"Step away from the door! Crazy woman exiting the room!" I shout and Carolanne's son laughs. Swinging the door exaggeratedly wide and banging it off the doorstop, we both hunch in fake-fright and giggle. "Don't tell your mum!" I march down the corridor with him following closely behind.

"There's plenty I don't tell her, and she's not really interested anyway", he says. This makes me turn and stop. He's taller than I thought, and we bang into each other. At maybe six feet or a little more, he's even taller than Jamie. My face reaches only up to his chest, which is broader than it should be surely? God, I really am *pissed*.

"Well, mums are a weird bunch. Trust me on that! I've learned to not have family around. My family are hundreds of miles from me. I've got used to it". My voice is cold, almost emotionless. Carolanne's son steps past me to open the door to the stairs.

"Pretty soon I won't see mine either. She wants me to join the Armed Forces, whether I like it or not". I can't see his face now, but he sounds emotionally exhausted by battling what is beginning to come across as a rather domineering mother.

Offering a little advice, I stop him on the landing. "Well, it's a chance to travel and get away. Way better than being stuck here! Try think of it that way". Ducking under his arm to start down the stairs, in this less than sober state, means my concentration is on not falling flat on my face, rather than the rather serious conversation.

"I suppose", he mutters and lets the landing's fire door slam behind us.

As we near the foot of the stairs, the noise of the crowded bar meets us, like a wave, and we both wince. "Mum throws a good party, so prepare yourself", he says and before I can answer, he pulls the door open and the deafening mix of laughter, squeals of "I've not seen you in ages!", "My round!" and "I love your hair!" over someone belting out Tom Jones on the Karaoke, hit me full in the face. Turning to see where

Carolanne's son has gone, there is just an empty space. I'm holding the door open alone now, and he's gone.

"Oi, Lola! Lola!" Carolanne's marching towards me, splitting the crowd like water. It's clear she's the boss, no one stands in her way for long, and a few people try to hug and kiss her as she strides past. "Let's get you a drink and find you a guy to shag!" she declares, taking my arm, and pulling me into the mass of bodies. All I can smell is alcohol, sweat and perfume and, for a second, I feel the need to be sick again. I've never been good with rooms full of strangers at the best of times, and this is certainly never going to go down as a "best of times".

Hoping Carolanne takes pity on how upset I clearly am, I try and brush off the idea of joining the party as best I can. "I'm actually just looking to buy a bottle of wine and head back upstairs, if that's ok?"

"Fuck no! You are staying. I've told the girls about you. "Girls" not being an operative term. They're as old as me and you!". She laughs so loudly a few dancers turn to look.

"I'm only 35 actually", I shout.

"Well, you look like shit!" she shouts back and shoves me towards a table, where two women and a man are sitting.

It's like they were waiting for me; they all turned in our direction. One of the women has an arm outstretched with what looks like a Gin & Tonic in her hand. The ice hasn't yet melted, and I can see the disco-ball lights are bouncing off it like sequins frozen in time inside the cubes. Suddenly, I'm thirsty.

"Go on then". Smiling and taking the glass, I go for the only empty seat at the table. A small, squat stool. The man seated next to me, leans over.

"I'm Oliver", he shouts, then clinks his pint glass against my glass. He doesn't make eye contact, but instead flicks a look at the woman who gave me the drink. Something passes between them. Two energies. She a warning, him an apology?

"Lauren", she says, smiling without showing teeth and not looking at him.

"Kay", the other woman nods at me, then takes a sip of her pint. Not clinking glasses with me, she watches me carefully and slowly drinks. It doesn't take a genius to work out that she's not happy I'm here. She's older than me, heavier, and isn't dressed as nicely. I've known her type and now I try to avoid them as best I can.

For the next hour, we try to talk over the noise of the party, but with my own stranger-status being obvious, I struggle to find the right things to say. There's a tension in the group, but as I get more and more drunk, my instincts slowly slip from my grasp, like paper straws falling to the floor.

"You haven't told us yet how you ended up here!" Oliver's words are blended together; I think he's even more drunk than me.

"I know!" I shout back and laugh.

"Would you like to go outside for a fag?" he shouts, but not as loudly. But I feel Lauren flinch.

"It's ok. I don't smoke!" I say, finishing my drink and starting to stand. He takes my hand, but under the table where no one can see.

"Neither do I", he whispers then winks. In a beat, he's tugged me down to his level, not letting go of my hand.

His breath smells surprisingly fresh and he's not that bad-looking. A flash of Jamie and Sharna having sex in the car I bought for his 40th birthday last year slaps me square between the eyes. Sitting down abruptly, so as not to fall to my knees with the sudden, shocking pain, Oliver take this as permission to lean forward and kiss me full on the mouth. Pulling back quickly before he puts his tongue inside, my shoulder hits Lauren's hip as she pushes past me, and heads in the direction of the toilet, *fast*.

Kay's staring at me, hatred coming off her in waves. She's not said much since I sat down. As she appears to be the oldest of the group I wonder if she's jealous. Looking away and embarrassed, even though I don't know why, I pull my hand from Oliver's, as I realise he's still holding it. "You shouldn't have done that. Whatever's going on is nothing to do with me", I hiss in his ear. He tries to kiss me again, so I push him in the chest and stand up, fast enough this time that he can't take my hand again.

"Night, then", Kay is dry and sarcastic. I don't reply but watch as she sits back in the booth, crossing her arms over what I now see are rather ample bosoms. She's bigger than I realised, at least twice my weight; not someone I want a fight with, verbal or otherwise.

"Night, Kay". I pick up my clutch bag from the table.

"Awwww, come on! Don't be a dick! I was only messin'!" Oliver wheedles and reaches for me again.

"Night, Oliver", I call over my shoulder, and start to push through the crowd.

Reaching the door to the stairs, which I now see is right next to the ladies' toilet, I consider going inside to speak to Lauren. Normally, that's exactly what I'd do. I'm always the people-pleaser, always the apologiser, always the fixer... "Fucksakes!" I push the door open and walk in, before I change my mind.

She's leaning over the sink and soundlessly sobbing. "Look Lauren, I don't know what's going on. I don't even know you guys! Carolanne..."

"It's fine. It's what he does. Don't take it personally. In fact, don't even feel fucking special. You are fresh meat, just like I was once!" Her words all bang together in a rush; it feels practised, or maybe so much the truth that she's said it too many times before.

"Listen, I've been where you are. Maybe even worse. I had no idea and I'm pissed and you're pissed and he's pissed. Fuck, everyone's pissed. Dirty, dirty, men!" I'm trying my usual humour to warm the situation up and make a friend. All I seem to do is try to make friends, yet here I am with none.

Looking in the mirror, over her shoulder, I look a mess. The meagre make-up has gone, I'm flushed, and my pupils are huge. "Who the fuck would fancy me anyway? Look at me. I'm like someone blew me up with a bicycle pump, let the air out fast and chucked me on a sunbed for good measure!"

She laughs and it's only the second time I've heard her laugh tonight. "Are you staying, do you think? Not at the party but here, in the village?" She blows her nose, and the words are muffled, but I understand them fine.

"Maybe. I'm in no fit state to make any decision right now. It seems nice enough and I'm... between locations. Looking for somewhere new to settle for a bit. Had a bit of a... bad time recently".

I don't want to tell her too much, oversharing as usual. The closer I get to people, especially other women, the more they seem to not want me close. Sometimes they even end up disliking me. My neediness isn't just with men, I worked that out years ago. I have attachment issues, apparently. Well, that's according to a counsellor, lots of Google searches and long, long, lonely nights reading about why abuse victims go back again, and again... "Here's my number, if you do stay on. I walk the Boscastle clifftops on Boxing Day. A sort of tradition. Come, if you want?" She's typing her number into my phone and not looking at me, but I can see how tense she is. She wants me to stay and it's a nice feeling. All the upset and drama of 10 minutes ago forgotten.

"I'll text you either way, ok?"

"Dirty, dirty, men!" She shouts after me in a silly voice, as I unsteadily navigate the strangely weaving stairs.

"Dirty, dirty, men!" I shout back in a fake posh accent. I can hear her laughing above the now-waning party, even as far as the first landing.

Pretty sure these stairs didn't move, left to right, earlier! It's like being on a boat! Giggling, it takes me almost five minutes to let myself in the room. Phoebe greets me, as though I'm just back from World War Three and I snuggle into her fully-clothed, for what becomes a 10-hour sleep of quiet, uninterrupted, blackness.

Listen to: The Pretenders – Angel Of The Morning

Chapter 5: White Water

The air is like knives on my skin; it is *absolutely freezing*. Not a cloud in the sky on the 26th December doesn't mean sunshine, it means ice-burn!

Lauren's walking next to me, wrapped up like a caterpillar, her dark blonde hair all caught up in the handknitted scarf wound tightly around her neck. I've opted for a beanie hat the sane colour of the slate-grey sea to our right. My long, padded and warm cream-coloured coat, zipped right up, has me joining Lauren in the mini-beast fashion show.

We started at Boscastle harbour and made our way up a steep footpath, to reach the long, flat path on the edge of spectacular cliffs. The views are breath-taking, even though the sky is grey and a cold fog hangs over angry ocean.

Never one for heights, I keep steering Lauren slightly to her left, so we're not so near the edge. Each time we find ourselves closer to the edge, my heart flutters so fast that my mouth goes dry. The anxiety disorder caused by Jamie and Sharna has me unearthing all sorts of strange phobias; phobias and fears that I never had, until The Toxic Twosome were part of my life.

Even before I dressed, I looked again today; I know shouldn't have. Like picking at a scab, I opened Facebook to see Sharna's unblocked me yet again. A deliberate "fuck you - see how I won", she's still trying everything possible to hurt and mock me. Now I can see her page, it's obvious they've been cheating on me for weeks, maybe months. Her stalking me was just one of her ways of eroding my relationship with him, so she could move from ex and side-chick to full-blown partner, *yet again*.

It was all for nothing. All the humiliation and sexual favours. All the money, the energy, and the tears. Oh god, the tears! It was all for nothing. No, less than nothing. Now I'm broken, unemployed and dirty from the inside out. I'm left in tatters. I wasn't in tatters when I met him, not by a long shot; I was *married*!

Shaking that thought off and realising I had nothing to go back to bar more and more humiliation, I texted Lauren to tell I was going to stay another day or so "at least until New Year". She replied within the hour, delighted.

Last night's Valium had worn off, but having a new friend made me feel just a tingle of warmth in what was now an absolutely freezing room. Even Phoebe's warm body against my hip wasn't doing much!

A little hungover, I'd wandered down to the bar to see if Carolanne or anyone else was around to help me with the heating system in my room. The bar was totally deserted. Wandering around the lounge area, adjacent to the bar, I'd spotted a cluttered noticeboard. Curious, I drifted over and was impressed by how much went on in this seemingly quiet little town.

⁂⁂⁂⁂⁂⁂⁂⁂⁂⁂⁂⁂⁂

Postcards, post-its and posters galore! Bake-sales for the Cadets in the next village. Knitting clubs. Gardening groups. Even Alcoholics Anonymous! The advertisements for local activities all boldly clamouring for attention on the slightly-dusty corkboard. "Not as quiet as it seems then!" I mutter, but stop as another flashback takes me by surprise.

"I've been going to AA for nearly 10 years now. Sober, clean, and a mean-loving machine!" His laughter seems to ring around the empty bar, and I see stars. "No one knows what really goes on in private. It's the quiet ones you want to watch", Jamie said when we first met. I hate his voice seeping into my head. Deep, calm, and careful, he always seemed so in

control and confident. So aware of himself, and his charm. So good at manipulating me.

I didn't even know I'd sat down. The memory of the lies about his sobriety took my feet out from under me. Putting my head in my hands and closing my eyes, I count to 10 and smooth my hair back. Now sitting on the wide window ledge below the noticeboard, I lean back and breathe in and out for a further 10 seconds, and count myself down.

I went to a local addictions support centre earlier this year. The counsellor, Dot, really helped me with understanding Jamie's chemical reliances, and how I could cope better with them. Initially, I had a few panic attacks when describing the disgusting things Jamie did when high, so Dot took me through some breathing exercises. They've come in handy but go no way to deleting the feelings or images that refuse to fade.

Jamie hated me going to the sessions with Dot. "They'll make you leave me, Lola! I'm going to prove how much I love and need you", he'd said as he deleted the charity's number from my phone, dropped it on the floor, then gently pushed me face down onto the sofa.

I'd been so relieved he didn't throw me out of the house in a rage, that the sex that time was different. I let him do something he'd nagged about for ages.

"Stop. Please stop", I whisper into the collar of my sweater. The smell of the wool was comforting but didn't stop me hyperventilating. I know I need to stop the flashbacks somehow; since I've left him, they're getting worse.

"Are you ok?" The familiar voice of Carolanne's son flicks my eyes open. Hastily pulling the collar of my jumper down and back into place, I'm red with embarrassment. Sat here muttering to myself, rocking and counting. For goodness sakes!

He steps out of the gloom and walks towards me, carrying a glass of water. "You're upset. Take this". It's in my hand before I can say no. I'd rather it was a gin. It's not even 10am.

"Thank you - I'm a weirdo", I blurt before I can think of anything else to say.

"No, you're not. It's a panic attack. They taught us about those at school".

Shit! He's younger than he looks. Fucking school! Mind you, he seems more mature and caring than that bastard at home. "Yeah - I've had them a while. Long story and not for your ears". I take a sip, close my eyes, and breathe deeply to stop myself crying again.

"I need to get on. Mum has got some temper on her if she catches me messing about".

I watch as he walks briskly out of sight. The room is dark, like most old pubs are during the day, but I shout "Thank you!" after him anyway.

* * * * * * * * * * * * * *

Now here I am, in Baltic temperatures and I do, actually, feel a bit better. "How long are you going to stay for? People come here for a visit and never leave. It's that kind of place", Lauren's rabbiting on.

I wonder if maybe she was one of those people. "Are you local then? Like from here?" I ask before I can stop myself.

"No. I came here for a summer job about seven years ago, met Oliver and I'm kind of stuck here, now". I wonder what she means by "stuck", but this time I stop myself from asking any more questions. Problem is, it leaves a space for her to ask about me. I'm determined to try and stay mysterious - not leave too much information behind me. Instinctively, I know She and He will want to ruin whatever goodness I try to build, wherever I do end up. They've done it before.

"It's a busy wee place though, isn't it? I can see how folk do get drawn in. Loads to do and folk seem really friendly". My words catch on the wind, so I have to shout the last two words. She frowns at my mild Scottish accent, but doesn't ask any more about my heritage. I cock my head, waiting for her to say more, but she looks away quickly.

"Yes - definitely friendly", she replies.

I open my mouth to ask where she came from if not local, but Lauren's already onto a different subject. "If you look over there, you can see all the way around the headland. We won't do the whole walk today; it really is too bloody cold and it's past gin o'clock!" In slow motion, she turns to me grinning, but all I feel is a rush of nausea as the world goes black.

"You drink too much, Lola". Jamie's voice booms in my ear. His hands around my throat, my feet aren't touching the ground. I'm desperately clawing at his wrists, trying to gasp even a little oxygen in. "Gin o'clock. Gin-o'clock. Fucking bitch!" He's raging in my face and spittle lands on my cheek. His breath stinks of vodka and coke, and there's a waft of tobacco as he leans in closer. "You should be in AA with me", he says slowly and carefully, as if he has an idea forming. Then he drops me.

"Lola! Lola. Jesus Christ! I don't know what to do! Lola!" Hands slapping my face. Different breath. Chewing gum and sweet coffee. I'm back home. No, I can smell grass and the sea. "Can you hear me?" I don't know who this person is, but it's not him at least. Opening my eyes, I'm blinded by bright sunlight and watch as a gull soars overhead.

"Fuck. I feel sick".

"You bloody look sick. You're a mad grey colour! What happened?!" she asks. I might look grey, but I feel as white as the sea froth I can see as I turn my head to work out where I am. A few feet from the cliff edge by the look of it. A surge of nausea gathers in my throat, and I thank god I didn't eat breakfast.

"Let's get you up and home. Well, back to the pub anyway. I know it's not home. But it'll do". She talks more than I do, this one.

"Yeah - I think that's a good idea. But let's just sit for a bit. My legs are jelly". This has happened before, only once but I know what it is.

****

"Blackouts and panic attacks can go hand in hand in extreme cases". My GP is taking my blood pressure and looks concerned. Initially thinking Jamie had finally managed to get his way and make me pregnant, I've rushed off to the doctors as soon as I felt I could walk straight.

"Is there anything going on at home that maybe has triggered this stress reaction?" The GP's sitting back in his chair and steepling his fingers in what I think, he thinks, makes him look mature and knowledgeable. More knowledgeable than a baby-faced practitioner with acne his mum dressed in too-short trousers, anyway!

"Nothing I can think of, no." I keep eye contact and my pale puffy face totally deadpan. I can tell he is trying to read me and work out if I am lying. But I don't even blink. In my head the answer was easy!

"Well, the love of my life dumps me at least every fortnight. When he lets me back into the relationship and his bed, I find dozens of texts and videos of him masturbating, and women doing the same back. The women and some girls are named after the different areas he works in in the local leisure centre and in his groups in AA. So lots of the females I've met. Do you know, I recently worked out he and I have maybe even had sex in the same places, and in the same ways, as he has with them. Oh, and by the way, he asked me to marry him last week and then yesterday he strangled me because I asked him about al his women".

"It seems strange that you are exhibiting severe anxiety and fainting, Lola". The GP looks in my eyes with a little torch and I wince. "If there are any other symptoms, such as dizziness, loss of taste or palpitations, please do come back

and see me. You don't look right at all! And the last thing we need is for you to have a nervous breakdown!".

Biting back the words *"I've not felt right in forever"*, I nod and put my coat on. *"Thank you. I will".*

****

Now, sitting on cold grass with a virtual stranger, overlooking the sea, I wonder if maybe I could just take a running jump off the cliffs into the water and forget the last three years ever happened. Forget my life ever happened.

I start crying as Lauren leads me away from the edge and gently sits me down, close to her for warmth. The tissue she found in my pocket, from yesterday's drive, is crusty. She comments on it which only makes me cry harder, realising how many gallons of tears I must have shed over a man who I missed and hated in equal measure.

"I don't know what's happening to me. I can't seem to just stay normal, or stable, or whatever I'm supposed to be! I-feel-useless-and-ugly-and-stupid-and-lonely-and-sad-and-angry-and-free-and-lost-and…"

The sobs take over again and she puts her arm around me. "Look - let's just get off the cliffs and go get warm. You don't need to tell me anymore and, by the looks of it, talking and thinking about it is knocking you sick!"

The pub's all lit up, as it was last night. Although not bustling and throbbing with people, most of the tables are taken, apart from the one I've realised Carolanne takes for herself and the other bar staff. Her usual magazine is on the seat, although she's nowhere to be seen.

Walking in, Lauren's hand tightens on my arm as we both spot Oliver at the same time. He's laughing hard with a group of men who I recognise from the night before. He doesn't turn to look at us, although one of the men makes eye contact with me and then nods at him, as if to signal our presence. Lauren walks a little faster and I'm a bit embarrassed as she sits me forcefully down at Carolanne's table. "Wait here, I'm getting drinks", she says and marches away, unbuttoning her coat as she does.

Taking my own coat off and pocketing my beanie hat , I watch as Lauren walks the long way around the bar, and looks towards Oliver as she passes him; hoping he turns to look at her. My chest tugs for my new sweet friend, as Oliver's back stiffens; but again he doesn't give her the attention she so sorely wants. Lauren's face burns and her shoulders droop a little as she reaches the bar. "Dirty, dirty men", I hiss under my breath as I reach inside a pocket for my room key.

I hadn't wanted to take Phoebe to the cliffs so had walked her on the beach earlier. Gesturing to Lauren that I was going upstairs to get her, I wave my keys and hold my fingers up to signal five minutes. Lauren smiles and waves, then turns back to the bar to Carolanne who's appeared as if from nowhere.

Skipping up the stairs is easier sober, that's for sure! I don't feel dizzy now, just thirsty. I'm not going to check my phone; triggering another panic attack would be stupid, as if haven't been anxious or sick enough already today. Walking down the corridor I can hear a gentle whining, and know that Phoebe's caught my scent and is desperate to see me. This time she'll be thinking I've been gone for days!

"You look hot today". Turning fast, I'm nose-to-nose with Oliver. He's followed me up the stairs, fast and light.

"Well, I'm busy as well as hot, thanks", I retort and start to spin away. He catches my elbow and, swift as a rat, is in front of me and blocking the door. Phoebe's whining goes up a notch and she starts scratching at the door. Panicking she'll mark the wood, I get angry fast. "Move. Now." I growl. Oliver has the good grace to look a little shocked. Yes, he needs to know that I'm not as soft as Lauren.

"Hey, hey! Just messin'!" He backs away and leaves a cloud of lager breath. I waft at it, making a show of how gross I think he is. "Cheeky bitch," he mutters and pushes past me, and I fall against the door frame. It hurts, but I don't react.

"Dealt with bigger and uglier than that, Pheebs", I whisper into her fur when she greets me, one key turn and five seconds later. She's so excited, her body writhes enough to tip me backwards onto the carpet; delighted at this new game, she takes the opportunity to lick my face far more than I'd usually allow. The salt on my skin, in my hair, is a second-hand treat for her.

"Right m'Lady, let's sort a wee feed, then a quick trot on the beach before we go to the bar, and you might even get a treat!" Phoebe steps backwards and jumps up on her hind legs like a small white T-Rex and I laugh; it catches in my throat as I remember how Jamie used to want a "treat" if I'd offended him in some way. Sudden oral sex, as he sat on the sofa, was *his* favourite *treat*.

I don't feel sick this time, but tears do promise to flow if I don't get the hell out of the room and back into the fresh air fast. Forcing the memory deep, deep down, two minutes later, I'm unleashing Phoebe in the car park and we jog the hundred yards to the beach .

Listen to: Shawn Mendes – Treat you Better

Chapter 6: Filth

Don't ask me how it happened and it's not what you'd expect. It's now almost four months since I fell into the bay here. Well, fell into this community!

Feet first, and barely even thinking about it, I just swam through the first few days and, taken by the tide, February came faster than I expected. It's left me feeling an occasional wave of panic, about how to stay afloat now my escape fund is draining away.

Bridgefell is one of those villages where no one seems to know the difference between Friday and Monday; every night, the pub is packed, and every day the little cobbled streets are busy. Even though it's not high season for tourists, it just isn't as quiet as I expected, or anyone would expect! I like the timeless feel of the place; the way everything is consistent, easy, and low drama. Love-bombed by my new friends (even Kay has thawed out!), I've started to obsess about how I could stay here, how to make it work. Well, for at least the Summer Season.

"What're your thoughts on a sort of cheese pie? Made with that local cheese... you know, the whipped one with herbs and too much garlic in it?!" I'm chewing a pen and making notes for my new boss, Jen.

"Up to you. You're good at these sorts of things!" She leans backwards out of the kitchen to look down the serving area to look towards the counter, where I'm standing with chalk in hand, writing a new menu.

"I do sweet, you do savoury. That's the deal, Lola!" she calls, and her face disappears again. I can smell lemon cake and something spicy, probably those hot cross buns she never seems to stop making.

I've worked here about eight weeks now, and *love it*. Jen is an absolute angel and the money, although not much, is enough for me to have a simple, fun, and low-stress lifestyle. In fact, I am daring to feel safe. The time has come to focus on getting better. After the peace of the last few weeks, I feel better. Not a lot, but enough. And it's all thanks to Lauren and Jen.

****

"Ohmigod ohmigod! I love Staffies! What's she called?! How old is she? She's gorgeous!" Phoebe's jumping, wagging, wriggling, and panting in a whirl of white and black, and loving every second of this new person's time.

"She's called Phoebe. She's four and yes, she is **gorgeous!**"
I laugh, even though I feel slightly awkward standing over this woman while she and my dog are both at knee level. It's a Sunday afternoon and the pub is in its only quiet phase of the day, between 12 and 2; just before the bingo starts. I've started coming with Lauren and, occasionally, Kay, even though money's started to run short now it's the middle of January.

Thankfully, the woman stands up to face me, and Phoebe huffs off in disgust, finding her usual cushion under the table. "I'm Jen. I run the vegan-sometimes-omnivore *café cum deli place down by the pier", she says breathlessly, hand outstretched. She's maybe my age, no older. My size but more tanned.*

"Wow! Where've you been!? That's some tan!"

Jen smiles and guides me towards the bar. Clearly, she's keen on a longer chat! "We have a place in Portugal. My partner, Louise, and I pop back and forth to run our place here, and have breaks over there whenever we can. We just got back home this morning. Come to think of it, you're new!" She tilts her head as if trying to work out who I am. " You are… thingy's niece? No… daughter!" She looks thrilled that she's half-worked out I'm not a total stranger to Bridgefell.

"Sorry to disappoint. I'm fully new but not a proper tourist. Been here since Christmas, but it's looking like I won't be here much longer. Money is running short". I don't tell her I'm also drinking too much and sleeping too little. I've managed to put a brave face on both for these last few weeks, purely down to denial, alcohol, and the lack of contact from Jamie and Sharna. Although I have had some number-withheld phone calls, and trolling on Facebook.

"You might be in luck, Lola!" Jen's waving at Carolanne and gestures for a drink. "So. What's your poison, Blondie?" This makes me smile and laugh again.

"Gin and tonic, or gin and bitter lemon. Whatever's going!" She turns to me when I laugh. Narrowing her eyes and pausing her hand, the beer mat she was waving stops in mid-air, and the silence shimmers between us.

"Are you ok? Like properly ok?" she asks abruptly. I've made a mistake! My laugh too sharp, or maybe I just seem... **desperate**. The lack of sleep has me on edge and, although my new pub-friends might not have noticed, this new person has. She's smart, older, has a business. She's been around. Shit.

"Ok. Well, job's there if you want it". Turning away, she bends her head as they start to whisper, and Carolanne flicks her eyes at me over Jen's shoulder. Unravelling my scarf, and looking for somewhere to sit, I dare to ask more.

"What job is it, Jen, if you don't mind me asking?"

"Working in my place. I need to open up for a few months, make some cash, and then Lou and I can bugger off back to the sun before the Summer season really kicks in here". She's still talking closely with Carolanne and doesn't turn around and I'm glad. The urge to cry and hug her is immense.

"Here, take this and we can have an interview in the corner booth ". She brushes past me then laughs, "Lola! I'm kidding. I'm not picky. If you can cook and be trusted with a set of keys, then the job is yours!"

****

So here I am, Springtime and more or less settled. Well, on the outside at least. Things are definitely better than they were - Jamie stopped contacting me about a month after I left. The begging turned to rage and threats quite quickly. I was in the midst of it when Jen offered me this job.

Sharing late night drinks and long cold walks, I've explored a little of Jamie's abuse with Lauren but less with Kay. To be honest, I am just so ashamed because I actually miss the evil bastard. I've had too many dreams of him appearing here in Bridgefell, begging me to come back, saying he'll fix everything. The dreams only differ when they are sweaty, whimpering, nightmares of him coming to collect me and immediately demanding sex. In all honesty, even getting to this point, almost April, has taken every ounce of energy I have.

"Ok. Well, I'll run a recipe up, make a test batch of mini ones, and we can maybe try them out later!" Scribbling down a basic quiche recipe, and then calculating how much of that whipped cheese to buy, won't take long. It's nearly 3pm and I've not had lunch yet. Not that I *want* to eat. My appetite still isn't ok, and it's not helped by the filth I get sent on my Facebook in particular, on a daily basis. Oh! The GP's warning of having a strange taste in my mouth has just reminded me: I must register with a doctor here.

Ever since the news broke "Roll up, roll up, Lola's single" both on Facebook and in the real world, my inbox *has been a target for a weird mix of anonymous messages* from women saying they cheated with Jamie while he was with me, men who wanted to cheat with me against Jamie, and a cluster of dirty, desperate randoms who aren't able to act in a non-sexual way.

I've become strangely numb to it. Let's face, it the whole relationship with Jamie was psychological warfare combined with what, to all intents and purposes, was sexual abuse. In darker moments, I wonder if I'm addicted to sex addiction.

To make sense of why I have rapid changes in emotions that have no grey areas, and a hunger for sexual contact, no matter how unattractive I find the person, I've done some reading. Apparently, the numbness with inappropriate compulsive thoughts is connected to disassociation. Basically, when a human being just has too much stress of the same type, she or he goes into a numb state where the body tries to protect itself by not reacting either way, or in the right way.

"It happens a lot in abuse victims, particularly sexual abuse and domestic abuse", I read to Lauren only last week, as we sat sharing a cigarette outside the pub, in unusually warm sunshine.

"Well, it's fucking filth!" she blurted, loud enough for an elderly gentleman sat two tables over, to shoot us a look of disgust. We'd laughed and scuttled inside, coughing and spluttering, but not loud enough that time, but we heard him tutting as we scurried past.

I'm ashamed to admit that I've replied to some of the dirty messages. I know, it's gross; but is it really *that gross*? Like, I'm single now, and if guys can do it why can't girls? In a weird way, I want to see what it was that made Jamie do it to me and all his exes. What's the attraction of juggling multiple accounts? Contacting and grooming complete strangers? Even messaging them all the same stuff, to get all the same sort of stuff back?

A few times, I've got drunk and sat alone at night, looking at old photos of Jamie and me. Going over and over and over *why* he would have this uncontrollable need to manipulate, use and abuse nearly a dozen women online, at the same time. Why would *anyone* do anything sexual with someone they didn't fancy?!

Most, if not all, of his targets weren't as slim or fit as me. Most were a lot older, and some were far, *far*, too young! The problem with these intrusive thoughts, though, is that anger sets in; and now my anger makes me do things I've never done before, except with Jamie. It makes me want to punish him when, really, I'm punishing myself.

Occasionally, a message from some guy, a mate of his, comes in or a guy from his AA group, and in a fit of revenge or misplaced sexual need, I reply. It snowballs; I say, and send, things I normally never would. And I wake up the next morning, the phone still in my hand, and I curl up in shame and cry.

I don't really know what's wrong with me - nothing that not drinking and totally deleting the last three years of my life wouldn't fix! Neither of those are going to happen anytime soon. And, frankly, my self-esteem is already so low, that it hurts no one but me to entertain the filth sometimes. I know he would hate it. Jealous and possessive, even when he was cheating, it gives me a dark, tar-like, thrill to sometimes send stuff back to these guys; each picture or sext, a knife to his throat.

Yes, I get carried away, yes, I've four or five on the go at the moment. But we'll never meet. They will never get to touch me, but I know he *knows* that I'm doing it. I feel it in my gut. The paranoia of a Narcissist is almost like an instinct.

I've read somewhere that they are excellent at what's called "Cognitive Empathy"; it's not like real empathy where they care, though. Oh no! It's like an ability to read and predict people's weaknesses, needs, and confidence gaps. From what the Narcissist, or other type of domestic abuser reads there, they craft themselves as the "solution". All the while, they know exactly what they are doing and what the end result will be.

By sexually grooming and abusing me, he knows fine well that I'm now pretty much sexually abusing myself, in my need to fill the gaping holes and heal the wounds that he created. I'm as promiscuous and unfussy as it's possible to be; a mirror image of him.

Yes, Jamie knows what he and Sharna did to me, and he knows what I'm doing to myself now. I'm not his first and won't be his last. The *thought* of hurting him with his own jealousy makes me worse. In fact, it's making me worse as the hate gets bigger and bigger; swelling and roasting and burning inside me.

The smell of smoke catches my nose. Spinning out of the dark fog of self-loathing, I twist and turn looking for the source of the fire. Black clouds are squeezing themselves slowly out of the furthest oven . "Jen!" I'm running towards the kitchen area, already knowing what I'm going to find. Jen's sitting in a chair in the corner, staring into space. Her hands are white with flour and lie palm upwards. The acrid smell of burning sugar and lemon are making my eyes water.

Wafting the smoke around with my hands, and coughing in the smoke, I reach my lovely Jen and start to shake her. She takes a few seconds to come back to reality. Then she smiles blandly at me. "Do you know where my purse is?" she asks. "I need to see where my purse is".

The signs of Jen's dementia were apparent as soon as I started working at "Have Your Cake & Eat It". She was obsessive about recipes, making me go over and over the ingredients, lining them up, double- then triple-checking the amounts. Initially I considered OCD, but I saw dementia in one of my Great Aunts growing up. I knew the signs.

Throwing myself into the café, and doing more than was needed to compensate for Jen's creeping illness, was just another way to hide from what was going on deep inside me, in the dark places we all hide from.

Jen's condition started to worsen about a month after I started, almost as if the disease could relax and spread now she had me to help.

Her older partner, Louise, seemed oblivious, and it wasn't my place to raise it; especially being new to the village and a very new friend of Jen's. I didn't want to upset anyone, and certainly wanted to stay out of trouble as best I could. My bad behaviour and bad choices were reserved for the privacy of my room at night.

"Come on you, let's get you out of here. Easy enough to clean the oven, and we can maybe close up for the rest of the day. Do you mind if I call Louise? I think you need to talk about this. You and I both know what's not right here". Guiding Jen out of the kitchen through the fire escape, I look up and see that a friend of Oliver's is parked across the street. He's eating the large, well-packed sandwich that I made for him earlier today.

"Robert! Can you give me a wee hand just now?" At the sound of my voice, he opens the Land Rover door and hangs a leg out, although doesn't stop eating. His face appears and splits into a huge smile. I think I see a blush, too! It's unsurprising he's still eating with a mouth full of food. My sandwiches are pretty legendary.

"Jen's taken a bit unwell and I need to go and shut the ovens off, and put the fans on. I don't want to leave her on her own."

"No probs. Gimme here", he rams the rest of the sandwich in his mouth and starts to amble over to us at an excruciating slow pace.

"Fucksakes gonna hurry up, Robert!"

"Ooooh, keep your hair on! Mind, you sound all Scottish now!" Fuck. In my panic, I've not watched what I was saying, and it's true, my accent is more Scottish when I'm afraid.

"Shut up and help!" I can hear him laughing even when I'm back in the kitchen.

We've chatted a bit and I know he fancies me - if that's the word, considering he's the same age as me. He looks older though; black hair sprinkled with icing sugar. Icing sugar and not salt because, to be honest, he's quite sweet. Tall, easily 6ft 2. A bit dim: he's no genius but seems a decent enough guy. The other night at the Easter Fair Dance, he got far too merry and stole a flower from one of the displays of fake flowers, for a competition managed by the local care home.

****

Sliding into the seat in front of me, Robert thrusts a big fake rose at me. "You're interrupting my pint, Romeo," I quip and hand the rose back. He pushes it back at me and makes deep eye contact. Admittedly, this is "a moment", but I am drunk and he is drunk, and I'm not a fan of roses. Well, not white ones made of a cross between plastic and paper, anyway.

"You're too nice for me, Rob. Don't bother trying to get in my pants."

"No, I'm not too good for you and yes, I am trying to get into your pants. And very fine pants they are, indeed!" He retorts, and thrusts the flower at me again.

"Aren't you seeing someone? That girl with the big buck teeth?" I'm handing the flower back, again.

"Nah. We broke up. She was mental. You're not mental, though. You're different." He sits back and puts the flower between his teeth which, to my annoyance, makes me smile and a giggle bubbles in the back of my throat.

****

"Oh, I'm different alright." I mutter opening each oven door in turn, and shutting them with a slam. I'm checking to make sure no other food is cooking, and turning them off. There are four ovens in Jen's bistro kitchen, including a little one she calls mine. Not sure why she does that, but it feels nice; like I'm special and I belong here.

Robert's my usual type, it's true. Tall, dark, not fat, and definitely not exactly a mastermind, but if he's as nice as he seems he could, maybe, have a chance. It's been weeks - no, *months* since I had sex. The thought burns my face. Jamie and Sharna will have been having sex; it's what he does. In the early days, sex, sex, sex. Fakes love and even lust, by taking a woman's body and doing what he likes, and making her think she likes it.

Jamie would absolutely hate it if I started dating anyone. With any luck he'll never find out because, if he did, it would mean that I'm not totally ruined; that there's something left inside me... something that might lead to plans, dinners, holidays... maybe even children.

Flicking the fans on, one by one, I'm starting to make my mind up. Turning back to the empty bistro, I can see through the big arched window onto the street. Robert and Jen are sitting on the short wall around the car park, and he has an arm around her. He's even sharing what I think is a chocolate bar. I watch as he breaks it into pieces and hands her one, then two, pieces. He says something and she laughs.

Robert senses me watching; he looks up and we make eye contact. He shrugs and makes a phone sign with his spare hand, and then grins at me. Something like attraction twitches in my chest; I look away, and step out of sight. "Please, don't let him be a dickhead!" I whisper, looking up at the ceiling in quiet prayer.

I'll clean the ovens tomorrow. Dear lordy, they are filthy! The smoke won't have ruined them, but they do need a clean. Right now, I think I'm owed a night out. Maybe I can even call it a date.

Listen to: Sia and David Guetta – Flames

Chapter 7: The Mistake

No, that wasn't a mistake like you think it was. Aye, it was a mistake, but not the way you'd guess. Or maybe you have guessed? If you think you have, you're still wrong. And those of you who are guessing right, I wish you *were* wrong. I'm rambling, but that's fair enough, considering I've drunk half a litre of gin, taken two Valium, and haven't eaten or slept in three days.

It's stunningly bright and hot; the sun's streaming through the window into the little room I rent from Jen, and I'm still freezing. Phoebe's asleep, as usual; we had a long walk along the shore at 6am. I prefer early morning as it's not just cooler, but there's fewer people to say hi and bye to. Phoebe's made friends with a spaniel called Joy and, I don't know the walker's name, but it's like she knows I don't want to chat. So, even when we meet at the same time each day, on the same pebbled stretch of beach, we just say, "Lovely day starting" and walk past each other. Nothing else said.

Last week the calls started; it's the same all over again. "He's mine. Leave him alone, old bag. You're a slut". Over and over the messages and texts shatter the mild peace I was starting to feel. It's a withheld number, just like it always is. Just like Sharna and her friends used to do. Robert says he doesn't know who it is. But I know who it is. I might be a raging alcoholic and suffering from the worst flashbacks you could imagine, but I know an ex's rage when I hear and read it.

Around and around the words and images go; all chased by sickness and suspicion. How can this be happening again?! I don't understand. I'm a thousand miles away and Sharna's still in my life, making me ill, and Jamie is still letting her. Is it *him*? Is it *her*? God, I don't know.

Finishing what's left in my glass, I check my phone. I see that Robert's messaged me. "Can I come over? I'm horny", it reads. I'm so, so sick of this. I like him, I feel even more than *that* for him, but this is suffocating. All these messages from men or women or something in between. Fake accounts, withheld numbers.

Drinking too much isn't helping now; not now it's all blown up again. I have this awful feeling of being watched too. Whenever I go out with Phoebe or Lauren, my phone and social media blow up. It's like whoever it is - although it's almost certainly Sharna - is able to track me and wants to ruin even the slightest nice time I am trying to have.

Turning the shower on, I know I need to sober up. It's Sunday and I'm meeting Lauren. She's worried about me, but obsessing over Oliver again; they slept together last week, and it's spiked in her this mad, needy air. I can smell it. She's just another me. "Get a grip, Lola!" I shout to myself, sat on the toilet, waiting for the water to heat up.

Jen's abroad again; Louise took her soon after the incident last month. Telling a woman her partner is ill, just on the cusp of a wonderful retirement, was heartbreaking. She was angry at first, shooting the messenger. "You're making trouble. It's not true. She's fine. You're a drama queen and exaggerating just to get attention, just like you want. Ever since you came here, it's all you, you, you!" Louise roared in my face.

Tears streaming down my own face, I sat there and took it as Jen simply took bank and membership cards out of her purse and laid them out fan like, counting them under her breath. "Nationwide. Co-Op. Boots. Nectar. Nationwide. Co-Op. Boots. Nectar".

"Louise, please stop shouting. Let me help. I had a charity job once where I was trained in the signs. I can at least help you get a diagnosis and some support, or even look after the shop while you go away. Some sunshine and rest, at least, is good for you both. It's never a bad thing, is it?"

She glares at me, opens her mouth to yell some more, and then drops her head and sobs. That sound as she keened, while her partner simply muttered "Nationwide. Co-op. Boots. Nectar…" in the background, made my chest hurt so much that I thought I was having a heart attack.

* * * * * * * * * * * * * *

Choosing to ignore Robert's booty call text for now, I step in the shower. The water pounds my head then shoulders, and starts to sober me up a little. I've been given beta blockers by the doctor. Anything to stop the relentless stampede of elephants in my chest at the slightest loud noise, ping of my phone, or ring of the doorbell of the house Jen and Louise have asked me to look after while they're away.

None of this makes sense; I should be better. Better than I was! It feels as though my demons have caught up with me, and eating me from the inside. It's like while I let my guard down and dared to hope for even a tiny bit of happiness, they've crept into my brain and soul. Like they are all hidden in corners, bent down panting, and waiting. Now that I'm beginning to like Robert, and making a success of the deli and shop while my friends are away, the monsters are crawling and creeping towards me, ready to take me over. To ruin me for ever.

Reaching for the shampoo, I notice a tremor in my right hand. "Look! Fucking get a grip. Have your shower. Go to the effing Bingo. See your friends. Keep trying with Robert". Yeah! I'm actually making sense now. Thank god for water!

Phoebe's sitting on the bathmat as usual, standing guard while I shower. "No worries, Pheebs. Mum's all good. Well, as good as Mum can be!" She Staffy-Smiles and I feel a little better.

"See you downstairs in 40; you can wait for sex. I'm busy" I reply to Robert once I've wrapped my hair in a towel and dried my hands.

"Awwwww", he replies with several aubergine emojis and red hearts, and it makes me smile. Initially I was terrified of letting a normal guy in and start a "normal" relationship. But it's been almost a month, and we've had no issues other than this mad female messing with us, who Robert insists vehemently is not Horseface the Ex. In fact I do, actually, really like him, even if he is a bit... laid back.

Jamie's fucked up my self-confidence, but I can't let him ruin me forever! Yes, the best thing to do is give Rob the benefit of the doubt. Those messages could be from anyone, especially Sharna! Men are simply idiots, and they confuse sex with intimacy. There's a saying about women having sex for love and men making love for sex or something; either way, it shows different genders have different agendas. Now there's a good name for a book... if I ever get around to writing one!

* * * * * * * * * * * * *

The bar has that nice busy but not crammed feel; I love a Sunday here. Maureen, who does the bingo, looks even more spray-painted than usual. Her hair doesn't move. Her skin is so wrinkled, she looks like someone once made her into a paper ball then unravelled her. She never, ever wears different shoes, always the same green wellington boots.

"Okey dokey, hokey kokey", Maureen yells into the microphone and all 26 of us in the bar wince. You'd think we'd be used to her dulcet tones by now!

"Here we go," Lauren whispers, and sips her drink. Even Kay smiles, and looks at me over the rim of her glass. Oliver seems a little uptight; he won't look at Lauren at all. I've noticed the tension mount bit by bit since I joined them 20 minutes ago. Robert has his hand on my leg, and I don't mind it so much now I'm a few drinks in. Yeah, Rob's a touch needy, but I prefer that over changeable, abusive, and vacant any day!

One thing that has me looking at her again and again, is Carolanne looks rosy and... puffed up... like she has a secret... It's disconcerting. She's not talked to me much today, or yesterday, actually.

Then again, she always likes to be the boss and it's more likely she has a new guy on the go, or maybe some gossip for us that she's saving for later; warming it up, practising how to share it for optimum effect. This idea tickles my chest; I resist shivering, and something akin to instinct rears its head. It's been a while but, since I left Jamie, my intuition has started to wake up, slowly but surely, and I'm not sure I welcome it. That dark, sticky, annoying feeling that something bad is coming.

Carolanne's son walks by, carrying a tower of ashtrays from outside. He catches my eye and nods. I wave cheerily back, but feel a pang of embarrassment for him; Carolanne has no qualms about insisting he wear an apron to "work" for her, even though he barely gets a wage and, more often than not, Carolanne is taking a break while Sam rarely does.

"I'm starting to agree with you, Lola. Leaving here and leaving mum to it might not be such a bad idea after all!" he said to me last week, when we stopped to talk on the beach. Sam started walking on the beach before work, soon after I came to the village. "I look forward to seeing Phoebe, and you always manage to give the right advice" was the excuse he gave when I jokingly asked how come I kept seeing him at the same time every day, even though obviously he doesn't have a dog!

****

Although blushing profusely, Sam is deftly avoiding eye contact and exaggeratedly making a fuss of Phoebe. It's pretty clear he's developed a full-on crush. Mind you, it's not uncommon in teenage boys to have a Mrs Robinson-type idea about one of their mum's friends, or a teacher! I'm actually flattered by Sam's attention. It's so different to the other men I know and have known. It's not sexual, or hungry, or needy, or jealous, or demanding.

Sam's talking again but, with his back to me, I can't make out exactly what he's saying. It strikes me that whatever he's saying, he's not keen on sharing, but is forcing himself to.

I touch him lightly on the shoulder and he turns to look at me. Phoebe glares at me in fury for interrupting her tickle session with Sam, and rolls back over onto her paws and sits to attention instead.

Sam stands and brushes sand off his hands. He looks like he's going to say something more, then changes his mind. He is sweet, and I feel bad that he is suddenly awkward, when he rarely has been before.

Jamie has made me feel so old, worn, and ugly, that male attention from someone, irrespective of age, makes me feel a little better about myself.

"You can do a lot better than Robert," Sam blurts suddenly, and I almost jump. It's like he's practised the sentence and my smile stiffens.

"What do you mean?"

Sam just steps away from me, pulls a weird face and walks away. Normally he walks me all the way to the pub, dragging his feet and enjoying our chats.

"Bye then!" I call, putting on a false affronted tone, but Sam doesn't turn and wave like usual. In fact, he speeds up! I watch as he awkwardly slips on the larger stones near the jetty, and jogs up to the street. I wanted to run after him and convince him that Robert is actually a really nice, loyal, guy. Instead, I'm rooted to the spot with worry that Sam is getting a bit too attached to me.

****

Oh! I've just remembered that. The creeping unease is managing to make its way past the four gins I've had and is snaking around my neck: tightening my throat and cutting off my blood supply.

Looking sharply at Carolanne, ready to ask her if something's wrong, I see she's no longer with us, and is hovering near her current fancy-focus and playing intently on her phone. She's probably sexting him, even though he's right by her. "My signature move", she told me soon after we first met. "Married blokes love it!"

Feeling suddenly cold and breathless, my stool squeaks on the tiled floor as I push it back, and all nearby faces turn to look at me. Making a "going out for a cigarette" gesture, I attempt at a weak smile and stagger slightly into the blazing sunlight. God, it's *hot*! Mind you, the thick warm air feels almost like a hug.

Opening my phone, out of habit, I start digging around in my bag for the packet of cigarettes I bought earlier. I've started smoking again. I always do when things aren't settled in my mind. Jamie isn't here to pull a face at me lighting up, while he deftly rolls himself a spliff. "We know what UR up to Slag", the text reads. It's come in while I've been in the pub.

Dizzy, I lean against the wall and close my eyes, taking deep breaths to try and settle the looming panic attack. "Who is doing this? Why won't they just leave me alone?" I whisper to myself and let out a sob. The urge to bang my head backwards against the wall tickles me behind the eyes.

"You ok?" Sam's voice is a little too close to my ear.

"Fine. Fine. Fine." I say, stepping away from him and knock into a wooden bench. The umbrella shakes threateningly, and Sam reaches across me to set it more firmly in place. I step out of his way and sit on the bench, hoping he'll sit with me. I want to ask about this morning, what he meant about Robert. I'm upset, frightened, and tipsy enough to be bold. The expectation that Sam has something important to say is firmly lodged between us.

"Sit down. Your mum's inside talking to that guy she likes. She won't peel herself away from him unless an earthquake starts". Sam smiles, but it doesn't reach his eyes.

"I don't want to cause any trouble but... well... maybe mum should tell you. You deserve better. You're a nice person, and it's not right - all this what's happening". Sam rushes the words out, as if chasing the fear away while talking. Not looking at me, and holding a dirty, froth-crusted pint glass in each hand, I can see he's shaking a little.

The sinking feeling starts at the top of my head and works its way down to my feet. On the way through my brain, the dread takes hold of my chest and squeezes the air out in a rush. Sam looks at me sharply, I think I must have gasped. I know what he's trying to say. I know what Carolanne knows. Neither of them need to say it.

With the perfect timing of a horror film, a yell across the street makes us both turn. "Sam! Where is he, then?! Come on! Fucking bastard better be hiding!" she shouts. The girl's marching towards us - no *past us* - and into the pub. The hot afternoon air is disturbed as she passes, and I catch a whiff of sweat, singed with something familiar. It's betrayal rage. I can almost see flames at her feet as she rushes through into the pub, looking for Robert. I don't think for one second, she's looking for anyone else.

It's Natalie, Robert's ex. I know her, but she doesn't know me. Robert described her to me before we started seeing each other and, typically nosey, I'd looked her up on Facebook. Startled by her horse-like teeth, so extreme it was almost a deformity, I'd laughed at him, cruelly demanding he tell me what the hell he was doing with her. Blushing, he'd replied she was a "psycho", and had got pregnant within weeks of them meeting years ago, so he felt he "had to do the right thing" and stay with her.

****

"Don't talk shit! You can be a great dad and not take the piss out of the kid's mum. Get that dealt with. Besides, I might be mean about her looks but, at the end of the day, it's cruel stringing her along. I've been where she is".

Regretting my nasty comments about her appearance, I'd laid it on thick for a while, as we sat on the pier with our legs dangling over the edge, a month before we first slept together.

The sun on our backs and toes in the icy, clear water, we discussed his predicament for hours. Robert was insistent that he wanted to date me, maybe even settle down.

"Well, I'd be gunning straight for you, Lola, if I did end it with Natalie. You know I fancy you!" Robert said, looking me straight in the eye before breaking into his typical wide smile. I'd nudged him on the shoulder, and he'd pretended to almost fall off the pier into the sea. I'd started to like him then, but had deliberately taken my time; wanting to do things right. Well, as right as I thought I was capable of.

"You fucking bastard! You've done it again, haven't you?! Where is she?!! Who is she?!" Natalie's yelling inside the pub. The background music that usually plays while the bingo is on has stopped, and a numbness falls over me.

Sam's staring at the doorway and is visibly shaking now. Poor kid. "Don't worry about it. I've handled bigger than her, love! It's Robert who wants to be worrying right now, not me or you. I can't believe your mum didn't tell me…" Tailing off as Natalie's yelling stops, I start to get up as she drags Robert from the pub, making him trip on the small step onto the street. He avoids looking at me, and she's too busy taking him to Hell to care who's watching.

Sam and I watch as she pulls Robert towards a small car across the road and, although we can't hear her now, the hissed instructions are clearly that he is to drive them home, so she can kill him there in privacy. I almost want to laugh, which is weird, because actually I want to cry. "Are you ok?" Sam's leaning over me. "Can I get you some water or ask mum for a drink for you?"

"I'm actually just going to sneak home". My voice is robotic; the shock has started to set in. I remember what it was like before, with Jamie. How can this be happening again?! This is so cruel. So wrong.

Not looking at Sam, I lift my bag and start to walk home. He makes a move to take my arm and stop me. I can't let anyone near me. I don't want him to see what I'm sure is going to happen next.

I can feel Sam watching me as I half walk, half stagger, across the street. Rounding the corner, and blessedly out of sight, I vomit gin and crisps into the shade and slide down the wall, and start to cry. This time, I do hit my head against the wall, and the pain makes me see stars.

I've taken two Valium, an anti-depressant, and am halfway through the bottle of gin I bought earlier. Earlier, when I had a boyfriend. Earlier, when I thought he was a nice person and maybe I was a nice person, too. Earlier, when I thought life was getting better, more normal. Earlier, when Carolanne was my friend. Earlier, when trust existed. Trust, friendship, and loyalty. How did I miss the signs? I've become what I most hated, the side piece. The slut. The homewrecker. The free fuck while a proper girlfriend sat at home. I hate myself. I should never have trusted him, or anyone, or myself. Is this my punishment for being too easy online? For trying to get my sex back? Trying to be like *him*, and learning why filth was preferable over fidelity?

Lauren's not picking up; she's probably with Oliver. The thought of them having sex makes me want to scream. What's wrong with everyone?! Why can't people just be normal?! Nice and normal!

Phoebe opens one eye, and wags her tail at the sound of me slapping my own face. A new game, perhaps. "Nope. Mummy's not well. No playing". She closes her eyes again and snuffles back into the pillows on my bed.

I'm curled up in the armchair by the window, overlooking the bay. Jen made the room she rents to me as nice as she could, even though it's small. "Small means cheap" I'd replied, when she showed it me, a worried look on her face a week after I started working for her. "I'll take it. Thank you." She'd been delighted.

"It helps me out too, really, as I hate leaving the deli *and* the flat empty when I'm away with Louise, so you're a sort of house-sitter and burglar alarm!" Hugging me, she stroked my hair and winked at Phoebe. Oh! How I miss Jen!

"Not one fucker in the world. Not one. Here we are again!" I shout, and Phoebe scuttles to her bed in the corner. Remembering Natalie's face, and Robert's obvious shame, I feel this crazy rage spread through my veins. He knew my situation; I'd trusted him with far more than I should have. I told him some things about why I was hiding away here in Bridgefell. Just like Jamie, I'd given Robert everything he wanted this last five weeks; all the sex he liked, any way he liked it. I'd paid for things; meals out, days out and even bought him some clothes.

I feel betrayed and violated all over again! God must hate me, or maybe there is no God. That thought makes me cry even harder. I've always had a solid belief system that, if you are good to your partner, have sex with them, and look nice, they won't cheat on you or leave you. It's not exactly a positive system, but it is one, nonetheless! It's almost as important to me as the other belief system I have, where there is good and bad, right and wrong. And, if you are a good person, good things happen to you and the world is a fair place. Utter shite. Total, steaming, shite.

In a world where "people" like Jamie and Sharna exist, there is no fairness. So again the belief system shatters. The sound of a heart breaking and self-esteem exploding is almost deafening. It leaves behind it a ringing in the ears, emotional emptiness and, worst of all, this huge, dark, void where hope and optimism once was. The shock is a killer - literally.

Almost crawling up the stairs, going over and over these facts, I whimper, slowly going crazy. Yet again. I think this time it's worse than before. Once is bad enough, I think. I've now been targeted, used, deceived, cheated on, and lied to, so many times, that I am what they say I am. Stupid, ugly, crazy, and a whore. Yes, I believe you now. I believe you.

Once in my room, I make a large drink, wash my face and slide down the wall, phone in hand. "Why didn't you tell me? You've been weird with me the last few days. He's your cousin, so you obviously knew about Natalie!"

Text after text, she receives them all but takes her time replying. Hitting me, hard, is the understanding that Carolanne is enjoying this. That *this* was planned. The strings between Robert, Natasha and I, all eagerly pulled by her. By God, I knew she had a dark side, a bad temper, and could even be cruel. I'd seen her with Sam, and even watched her bar punters from the pub who she took an irrational dislike to. I've seen her drop friends when it suited her, too. The edgy, nervous, atmosphere in the group isn't caused by Lauren and Oliver's toxic romance. It's Carolanne! People are afraid of her! But why?

Easily accepting some responsibility, I think I always knew she had a nasty side. But this, today, was startling. No, not today! She's been planning this, for days, maybe weeks! Maybe since Robert and I first got together! Why, though? I've never done anything to her! I've tried so hard to be friendly, and settle in here. Tipping the glass back, my eye catches my phone flash as Carolanne finally replies.

"Blood's thicker than water and, let's face it, you are no angel, Lola. Now fuck off. I'm busy", was the only response I got. Dropping the phone to the floor, I scream in rage and hurt before storming downstairs to the kitchen for ice.

I fall a few times going down the stairs, but don't feel it. A full on hot-mess, I am well on my way to something disastrous. A sore leg means nothing to the impending humiliation I'm going to have to face now; in this small place where I've tried to make a home.

Unsteadily making my way towards the bathroom, I can feel my old friend, self-loathing, is back. She has her arms wrapped tightly around me; it's hard to breathe or to stop the movie-reel of pictures and memories, none of them nice. Hatred for everyone, ever, swiftly follows her through the door. I'm not well, but now I don't care.

There's no point trying to have a normal life because no one's normal. No point trying to have a nice life because no one's nice. Oh God, I feel so ruined and dirty. I don't want to kill myself; I want to kill everyone else. The rage is different this time; maybe I'm too broken to feel things normally.

As I start running a bath, my phone pings. It's a message from a number I don't recognise, probably that Natalie again. It's all the same as last time. Just more intense and fast-tracked. For the last two hours I've had 15 messages from the number, calling me an "old tramp", "slag", "whore", "homewrecker" and, even, fat and ugly! Although, having seen her in real life now, I'm actually slimmer than her. But yes, she's right. I am older. A hundred years old. So many lies, each a line on my face, and a scar I'll never heal. My eyes are puffed with the things I've seen that I can never un-see. The bags literally hold onto the horror, like luggage. Maybe that's why they are called "eyebags"? Who knows?

Typically, I get the threats and abuse while she lets him back between her legs, and they carry on all happy families while I curl up in humiliation and horror. Stupid, needy, obsessed bitch; plenty of them everywhere, just like I was. My thoughts are vile, but I don't care.

The phone pings again and, this time, I'm ready to fight back. I made that mistake in the past and it only ever got me in trouble. But now I'm tired and humiliated, and ready to bring some of my own bile and hate to the party. Closing my eyes, I take a breath. Lip curled in disgust, mouth full of words as evil as I can muster, I read the message again.

"Just checking ur ok. It's Sam. I got your number off Mum when she told me to come and drop off that Top last week. Sorry. I can come over if you like? Do you need anything?".

Shaking my head a little to clear my thoughts, and reading the message again, there's a tingle of unease but it's not strong enough to stop me replying. Fuck it. Fuck everyone. I'm going to do something really bad and make myself feel better; my choice, my control, my life, my body. I'm not ugly or old or unwanted. I'll show *you*.

Listen to: Billie Eilish – Bad Guy

Chapter 8: The Drowning

"When can I see you again?" Sam's text reads. My heart's in my throat. It shouldn't have happened. What the hell was I thinking? No, not thinking, doing! I'm going to jail. *I'm going to rot in jail!* It's taken him no time at all to expect more of me. Fuck, *I* need to expect more of *me*!

"It can't happen again. I'm really sorry. I shouldn't have let you in the other day. Please don't be angry. Your mum will kill us both". He reads the message, I can tell, because I blocked him on my phone the morning after. Now he's contacting me through Facebook, and seems to be online every time I am, although from his page I can see he's not active in public.

Like most guys with an infatuation, he's most likely watching my page and waiting for me to message him. The waves of guilt for what happened, and shame for myself, wash over me again and again, and I feel like I'm drowning.

First thing in the morning, the fear hits me; last thing at night, I cry in remorse desperately trying to work out how the hell I ended up like this, sleeping with a boy turning 16 tomorrow.

Carolanne's cool with me; nippy even. She doesn't know, of course, but since we argued over her loyalty to Robert, and the nasty way she set up the ambush at the pub, we've spent the week dancing around each other. I'm desperate not to make an enemy of her but, at the same time, I am deeply upset by her behaviour.

In dark moments, fuelled by alcohol and anger, I think I deserve my secret this time. And it serves her right for being so bullying and cruel. This doesn't last long though; it's not the real me. I can't justify Sam and me. Not ever. No matter how hard I try and, actually, I don't really want to. If I try and excuse what happened and blame anyone else, I just end up like Jamie and Sharna. Being like them makes me have thoughts of dying all over again.

Confusion and sleeplessness has me in a deep state of denial for how bad The Mistake with Sam really was, but the fear has me experiencing daily panic attacks and horrendous nightmares about being killed in prison, and Phoebe being torn from my arms, whining then barking in fear.

Waking from these terrors, I cry into my pillow and beg for a way out; some way to go back in time and reply to Sam's first text, "No. It's ok. I'll see you tomorrow".

I've hidden myself away this last couple of days, and it's making people suspicious. Lauren finally came out of hiding with Oliver, pleased as punch she'd got her wicked way with him. Manic voicemails from her, "This time it will be different! This time I think he's going to love me properly! Come and meet us in the pub. It's Wednesday! Karaoke!"

I've replied only once to these excited and happy texts, with "I'm embarrassed about the Robert thing. Need a bit of time to sort my head out. Let things die down".

She called again a few times then, seemingly bored by me, or distracted by her obsession with Oliver, I was left alone. As a result, I've done nothing but sneak out early morning and late at night to walk Phoebe, or nip in the car to the next village to go to the off-licence.

Sam's messages with sad emojis; little blue tears and big round yellow faces do nothing to calm the turmoil and fear. He actually likes me and genuinely wants to have some sort of relationship!

****

To clear my head, I've started sea-swimming again. It's easy to avoid people, almost a mile out into icy cold water and the exercise is such hard work, I can forget my thoughts and simply take stroke after stroke and make kick after kick.

This is my third time out on the water, and it's getting easier. I met Jamie when I started swimming at my local leisure centre. Under his watchful eye, I went from six awkward laps, to over 100 each time I swam. The smell of chlorine now makes my IBS flare up, and even a flash of a lifeguard costume gives me the shakes. So, as a result, I secretly bought a wetsuit with a plan to sea swim wherever I ended up once I left him. I sea-swam and enjoyed diving as a teenager, and this takes me back to my teens.

Cutting through the light surf, I round the coast and prepare to turn back at the same point I always do. I've come out early today, as I plan to go to the doctors later. It's time I sorted my head out and prepared to either confess or leave. But leave in a healthier way than I arrived!

Men shouting and laughing catches my attention, and I stop swimming and tread water, and take my goggles off. About 100 yards away is a small fishing boat. It's familiar. I've seen it moored up on the beach at Boscastle, and once in our bay here in Bridgefell.

The sun isn't fully up, so the boat still has lights on, and the men aboard appear to be wearing head torches. Their laughter echoes that of the gulls who have yet to rise for the day. One of the men looks a lot like Oliver.

My chest tightens in panic. What is Oliver doing out here at this time? And what are they hauling up? Then Robert appears. I know it's him: I recognise that walk, and those familiar red overalls and goofy beanie hat he wears. The yellow and white stripes put me in mind of a comic character, and I've told him so many times before.

I swim backwards but keep my eyes on the boat and the men on it. In the darker parts of the rocks at the foot of the cliffs, I can rest a little yet still stay afloat. My body is cooling now I'm not swimming, and I know I need to leave soon, or I'll get too cold to move, and that is dangerous. Very.

The bell on the boat isn't ringing like it should when the boat sways on a choppy sea. I wonder if they have taken it down or taped it up, so they can be almost totally silent out here?

The sun is coming up and will soon shine directly on me; my wetsuit has a neon blue stripe down each side, and although my swimming cap looks dark now, rock-like even, once the sun or any light catches it, you can see the girly sparkly bits in the rubber. "Fuck!".

"Last one! Then home for brekkie! Good job, lads!" Oliver shouts and the men reply, although I don't quite hear what they say. Robert shouts something, but all I hear is "Sunday". I think they are repeating this, whatever this is, on Sunday. I think I may well want a swim that day, same time… too.

Two weeks later, and I'm driving back from the shops. "Fuuuuuuck!" I yell and slam my fists on the windscreen. My phone lights up. "I'm 16 now, so it's ok", a message reads. "No Sam. Honestly. Don't be upset or angry with me, but I really can't", I reply later, once a firm but kind message comes to me. More emojis from him, but I ignore it and go offline.

Today, I feel a little better, but that's only because I've come up with a plan of sorts. Walking towards the doctor's surgery, I falter a little and stop dead, a few metres from the door. How the hell do I tell the doctor what I did? How is there a way to explain it? I can't go to jail. People like me get killed, or worse, in jail.

I can't lose my Phoebe, my baby; it's a fate worse than any death. Breaking out in a cold sweat and feeling like I'm walking on a boat, the early signs of a panic attack start up. Leaning against a car, the hot metal burns the bare skin at the bottom of my spine, and I yelp and leap away. The pain has filled my eyes with tears.

"Cut me a break, please, will you?" I whisper, looking up at the sky. Don't know why I'm bothering; it's Hell I'm headed to now anyway, and the thought terrifies me. Not churchgoing but spiritual, and certainly a believer in Karma, I've tried to live my life right, and now here I am. I've done something unforgiveable and shocking and can never, ever, take it back.

It's never going to happen again; never. I knew that as soon as I woke the morning after. Once it hit me, what had happened, I knew no matter what that this had to be my rock bottom, and I had to save not only him from whatever upset I'd undoubtedly cause him, but my baby needed me to sort stuff out, at least for the time-being until the police knocked at the door. She deserved better and so did Sam.

"Do you have an appointment?" The receptionist's face is familiar, but not enough for a name to pop into my head.

"Yes, I made it last week. I've only been in the area for a few months. I don't know if it was you or the other receptionist who said it was a Dr Nigel Cafferty, or McCaffery, or something." For some reason, my throat squeezes and I want to cry. For this lady, with the big round face and bouncy perm, to hug me tight and tell me she'll fix it. The sense of panic is overwhelming. Holding onto the reception desk for dear life, I know I look sick. *She has no idea how sick I am.*

"Yes, you got the second one right. It is McCaffery". She emphasises the R in her lovely, rounded, Cornish accent. "Have a seat; we're running behind a bit today, but shouldn't be too long". She nods towards the last remaining seat in the corner of the waiting room. While walking slowly towards it, I try to avoid making eye contact with anyone, but fail spectacularly when I spot Kay, in the seat opposite the one I now have to take.

We've never been close, but she's a common fixture in the group of people I most often spend time with, in the pub and around the village. For some reason, we just never quite clicked and, with Lauren being my closest friend, then Carolanne, I didn't go out of my way to be pushy with Kay about getting any closer. The feeling that she just wasn't "the type" for bezzie mates was always there. Sometimes a whisper that she was judging me for being here, alone, and a bit "mysterious", tickled my ear, but I brushed it away and focused on trying not to be judgemental or paranoid.

"What you in for, then?" she blurts, slapping the newspaper down on the floor between her feet. Folding her arms, she waits expectantly. Clearly, I don't look so ill that I deserve a bit of privacy. How do I respond? Feels rude to say, "None of your business" or even "I'd rather not say". Desperately trying to think of something takes me so long that she speaks again. "I'm in for some tablets for my mental health. Reckon I might ask for counselling again, actually". Speechless at how frank she's being, and equally relieved that she's taking about herself, I try to smile in what looks like warmth, not relief.

"I'm in for something similar, actually."

"It's good here, things usually move fast and, because it's a small place, folk tend to not come and talk about stuff like this, as they don't want it getting out that they're nuts". She makes a circular, swirling sign with her finger against the side of her head, indicating the old gesture for "crazy".

"Yeah, well, I'm crazy for sure, so maybe this time they can fix me once and for all". Again, that awful drowning, suffocating, mix of feelings like I want to wail, and confess, and cry, and beg for forgiveness and help. Stuffing the words down so hard my stomach hurts, I make small talk with Kay for the next few minutes until my number's called over the Tannoy.

"Catcha later!" she calls after me, as I walk towards the smiling doctor, holding his door open.

"Erm, yeah. Bye", I say without fully turning. That's the nicest she's been since I met her! Weird? Maybe she's just a one-on-one person rather than chatty in groups, and our table in the pub can get a bit boisterous. Maybe I've made a new friend. God knows, I need one.

Lauren's now fully hooked back into Oliver, and Carolanne's not best-friend material; not at all. Poor Jen's deteriorating, but she's now abroad again, anyway. Resolving to make more of an effort with Kay the next time I see her,

I walk into the doctor's examination room and get ready to tell my story without really telling it at all.

Twenty minutes later, I'm practically running out of the surgery, desperate for a drink and to forget everything I just said. Going over what He did to me; what She did to us and then me, has made me feel so sick, I think I might throw up. I'm going to feel ill, really depressed now for a few days. These conversations always trigger proper dark periods that no amount of booze, blokes, and baths can ever shift. Regretting coming, and panicking about how to get through the next few days, I'm not watching where I'm going and bang into someone as they open a car door to get out. It's Kay.

"You're in a rush!" she shouts as I step back and start to apologise. "You look rough, too! All clammy and sweaty!" She starts to laugh. It's a bit cruel but, then again, I'm not in any position to consider what is and isn't cruel anymore.

"Hate appointments like that. All the talking, history and upset. Just triggers me and sets me off to be honest". My hands are shaking, and I actually smell of sweat and now, I think, stale alcohol. Shame burns my face, then spreads down my neck. Suddenly, it's just all too much and the floodgates open.

"Jesus Christ, Lola! You're normally so together! Get a grip! It can't be that bad! Whatever it is, you can get over it. We all do in the end. These are just blips. Meds and meetings and back on track!" She's chirpy but it only serves to make me sob harder and louder; she has no idea. I'll never get over this and, maybe, neither will Sam.

His face comes into my mind's eye. How happy he was leaving my flat. I'd watched from the window as he skipped off down the street and around the corner; lit up by the streetlight, he even looked like he was walking taller, straighter; all happy with himself. He turned around before disappearing from view, and waved, knowing I'd watched him leave.

"It doesn't matter. I just need a drink and a shower. Don't worry about me. Still waters run deep." She steps back and frowns at the last sentence. I'd said too much. Fuck!

"Sure, no probs. But if you ever need to talk, or come with me to a meeting, you can. Here, take this. My doctor gave me a leaflet, but I went last year, so I don't need the contact details".

She puts a shiny, brightly-coloured bit of paper in my coat pocket and then, out of nowhere, roughly hugs me. Taken aback, I just stand and gawp as she gets back in her car and spins the tyres as she leaves the car park. She toots her horn, and I half-heartedly wave, unsure what just happened.

Driving home, it hits me hard that I can't avoid the pub for much longer; there's only so long I can be seen to be mourning that rat, Robert. Carolanne hasn't gone out of her way to see how I am, but Lauren says she's been asking where I'm buying my booze. Typical Carolanne, that rough, half-hearted, compassion that I've had to get used to. I've never known anyone like her before; manly almost, and yet man-mad. We're not as close as I thought we'd be when I first came here. Lauren's gentler, intuitive, and caring nature drew me to her, and away from my neediness towards making a relationship with Carolanne, and I'm glad.

In a strange way, I'm afraid of her; not just now I've slept with Sam, but before that. I've heard rumours that she's not just got a temper, but form for obsessing over anyone who crosses her. That reminds me, I need to make sure that Jamie and Sharna haven't unblocked me, or set up any more fake accounts. The last time I looked he'd dumped her again, and his profile displayed yet another blonde, startlingly like me, but artificial.

She will be on the warpath again, looking to fixate on me again, most likely she's dumped like trash again. Making it all my fault, like it always seemed to be. She might even think he's going to come looking for me, revisiting the rotting corpse. The thought makes me shudder and, yet again, imagine myself dead and gone, hanging from a prison cell ceiling, the wails and shouts of women echoing over and over as my life slips away.

"Fucking hell! Why did I do it?! *What's wrong with me?!*" I shout and the car swerves a little towards the last ditch before the village comes into sight. Slowing down, patting Phoebe, and taking deep breaths, I turn into the pub car park. It's busy, the early summer weather's attracted a new swathe of tourists and, with it being Saturday, today's change-over day; they're absorbing as much sun and alcohol as possible, almost as though it's going to run out before their holiday even starts.

Carolanne's weaving between clusters of revellers and picking up empty glasses wherever she sees them, but not bothering with pleasantries. She's always been a bit grumpy but, today, she looks thunderous. My heart pummelling the back of my throat, I get out of the car but leave Phoebe inside with a bowl of water and the window open; it's too busy for her, someone will step on her paws.

"Where the fuck have you been, bitch?!" She shouts as soon as she spots me. I'm used to it, it's her way of saying hello. In the beginning she was nicer but, comfortable with being a bit of a bully to me, she's settled into it with ease.

"Not well. That Robert thing sent me daft, as if I wasn't already fucked up". Trying not to cry, I watch as she grabs a tray and hands it to me.

"Give me a hand. Sam's away to a mate's for the day, and left me right in the shit."

Glad of the distraction from actual, real, conversation, I start to clear the tables she hasn't of plates and glasses. "I've not got long. I need to open Jen's place for an evening shift. It's been closed all day, and I've food prep to do." I don't know why, but she's managed to make our friendship all about her, and I'm on eggshells most of the time, just like I was with Him.

I've let it go a bit too far, and Sam's nothing to do with it. I'm just so used to pleasing people and trying to keep the peace, I've missed where she started to be really quite mean and even cruel. Setting up that drama with Robert and Natalie might just be the final straw. "Fucksakes! Don't be a cow!

Help me out as long as you can. Always moaning, you are!" she says, storming into the pub.

One of the drinkers looks at me and raises an eyebrow, as if to ask why I put up with being spoken to like that; to be honest, the answer is too upsetting to give. "She's always like that, it's why I don't work here!" Trying to laugh, I choke on it a little, and carry on collecting from the tables to hide the blush that precedes tears.

A few weeks ago, she was actually quite nice to me, although at the time I was helping her clear her own flat out. "Here, you have this. He's not going to need it now; he's outgrown it so much". In her hands is an old football shirt; the regional team that I half-support, now I live here.

"Ok - thanks". Quite pleased with her kindness, I put it on over my clothes and she laughs at how well it fits.

"You are a tiny, skinny, bitch, Lola!" She calls, walking away to the next room to get more binbags for the huge amount of stuff she's hoarded over the years.

Then her voice changes, although I can't hear what she's saying. It goes up a few notches, and I recognise the tone she uses for berating Sam. "Come and look at this! Fucking disgusting he is! Lola, get in here!" My heart fluttering and already thinking that this isn't right, I walk towards his bedroom, which is off the living room.

"I don't think I should be in here, it's not nice. Lads like their private space". My voice tails off as I see Sam standing, slightly stooped, in the corner, mortified that I'm here; a witness to his mother's room-shaming. "Come on, let's go and finish this clear-out. Let him sort his room himself, Caro". I try to tug her arm and pull her away from what's making me cringe more than Sam, although that's unlikely.

"Get this place sorted. Now. It stinks. Dirty bastard!" She yells, waving her arms about; he flinches like she might hit him. I wink at him over his mother's shoulder and his mouth twitches, but he daren't smile. Luckily, Carolanne's throwing his duvet off to expose his bed, and doesn't see our exchange.

"Filthy wanker, you are!" *She's still shouting and this time, I'm not so patient.*

"Carolanne, you can't speak to him like that in front of me. You're embarrassing him and me. Now, get out of the room and come with me, or I'm going home!" *I've never stood up to her before and she turns around to glare at me, huffs and puffs, and pushes past me to leave the room.* "Tidy the room yourself and then she can't complain, Sam." *I whisper.*

"All she does is complain and shout at me, I can't do anything right", *I hear him mutter, before backing out of the room and quietly closing the door.*

Remembering this for the first time means that yet again I manage to flood the huge café sink and only realise once my stockinged feet suddenly feel wet. Crying, and drying the floor with paper towels, I don't hear the door open. "I need to talk to you, to say sorry". It's Robert.

Whipping up, nostrils flaring, and ready to fire off as many insults as I can before he leaves, I stop when I see he's holding a bunch of flowers that look like he's picked himself. "What do you want?" is the best I manage; already crying and embarrassed, the energy for a fight isn't in me. No more fighting. No more tears. It's only got me in trouble so far.

"I should have told you about Natalie. I never really broke up with her. She's a complete nutter and you are just the opposite, and I couldn't work out how to fix it. Before I knew it, I had a thing for you, then with you, and it all just rushed away from me."

He's babbling and looks like he might even cry. I'll give him his due, he's more of a man than the bastard I left at home. Cheat yes, but cruel and gutless, no.

"Look, I can't get involved in another situation where your ex, or whatever she is or isn't, can make my life a misery. I told you enough to know why that is. I'm a mess right now and your life is a mess, and she's wild as fucking rabid dog. I'm not getting back with you. Not a chance, Robert. I can't do it".

The last few words catch in my throat and Sam's face looms into view. Him waving happily in the streetlight.

"But we could keep it a secret?" he whines, and I find the energy to summon enough anger to snatch the flowers, slap his face, and tell him to leave.

"You're all the same; filthy, dirty, lying, cheats who want to have their cake and eat it!" I scream and then a crazy laugh escapes because we're here, in a shop called "Have your cake and eat it"! Robert backs out of the door as fast as he can manage; my lunatic laughing's scared him. "Don't fucking speak to me again!" I yell, as he jogs down the path towards his Land Rover, parked in its usual spot outside the pub.

Instead of putting the flowers in the bin, I take small sprigs and fill the bistro's table vases with them, slowly, one by one. I've always loved flowers, and it's not their fault. They're a pretty mix of pink and blue, it takes me back to the last time Lauren and I took a walk to the cliffs. "I'll text her later", I promise myself, and go back to drying the floor. I'm now really late to open.

A few days later, I pluck up the courage to go to the pub; it's a Friday, and busy enough that I can avoid too many long conversations about where I've been and, even worse, how I've been.

****

Kay, Oliver, Lauren and I are at our usual table and tonight, Carolanne's with us. Sam keeps looking over at me, but I'm refusing to make eye contact. I don't want any sort of atmosphere between us to get picked up. Paranoid, drinking even more than usual, and trying to adjust to the medication the doctor gave me last week, I'm barely holding it together. In all honesty, I'm scared of how ill I clearly am. Yesterday, I even considered leaving. Just packing up the car, shoving Phoebe in, and running. Yet again. Remembering this makes me want to scream and cry at the same time.

My phone pings, but I don't look. The immediate gut feeling is that it's Sam makes my throat burn with bile. "Why aren't you looking to see who that is?" Carolanne shoots me a look of disgust at how weak, or weird, she thinks I am today.

"Not in the mood for drama, and seeing as you lot are all here, bar Robert, it doesn't take a genius to know who it is", I shoot back, with more anger than I expected. Taking my glass, and heading for the bar, I don't wait for Carolanne to hassle me further. It's becoming clear she enjoys dramas, especially when she manufactures them.

Going to the furthest end of the bar where it's quieter, I open my phone. "Please talk to me. I want to see you again", the message reads. I was right, it's from Sam. "No - friends only. That's it", I reply quickly, even though my fingers are shaking. Sam comes out of the kitchen and starts to walk towards me. Shaking my head forcefully, I back away and, just before turning, see how his face falls. The guilt spiking my chest is horrendous, as I make my way back to my seat. I've not just done something illegal; I've hurt his feelings. *I hate myself.*

"Where's your drink?" Kay asks, her face even more lined now she's confused.

"Aye? Where'd you go?" Carolanne's put her glass down and is staring straight at me.

"Got yourself a bloke on the sly, have you?" Oliver asks, smiling even though his eyes are cold. It's no secret that he's still got a thing for me, but he's hidden it well since getting back with Lauren.

"No. I'm just not well at the moment and getting forgetful. Doc say's it's stress."

"Well, watch yourself because my Sam's smitten and if you were younger, I'd let you marry him!" Carolanne crows and throws the rest of her pint back. My heart stops. There's a few beats of what feels like complete silence, in the centre of the busy pub, then the rest of the table laughs along with her.

"Obvious as anything he has a crush on you!" she says as she walks away, taking the table's empty glasses with her.

"Pffffft!" Oliver huffs and follows her, roughly pushing Lauren's hand off his knee. She looks hurt and her face starts to crumple.

Simply for something to say to stop the landslide, I blurt "We've not had a walk together in ages, want to go tomorrow?"

Listen to: Sigala and Ella Eyre – Came Here For Love

Chapter 9: Green-eyed

"There's something I want to talk to you about". Lauren's voice is even more tentative than normal. Since getting back with Oliver, she's retreated into herself whenever he's not around and only seems to light up when he's in her eyeline.

"Sure, go ahead". I'm pretty sure it's about him, he's all she talks about anyway, and I'm happy for the distraction.

"Someone messaged me a few days ago saying you were seeing Oliver, behind my back". The words hit me full force and yet don't make sense.

"What? I don't know what you mean. No! Never!" Stopping dead on the little path we must have walked a hundred times by now, I grab her hand to make her stop walking and look at me.

"It came from Facebook. Some woman called Celia or something like that. I blocked her as she just messaged on and on about what a slut you are, and how you ruined her life and took her man". Over and over the waves are crashing in my head; it's Her. I knew this would happen. She's found me and it's all started again.

"No. No. No, Lauren. I promise you. I swear on my life, I've not been near him. I didn't tell you, but I do get a feeling he's a bit of a sleaze... he was... pushy with me, when I first came here, but that was ages ago. I know who this woman is. She's the mad ex-person who my ex has this toxic mad thing with". Pleading with her, I don't blink as I watch her take this in and summon up belief in me. No, in Oliver, her precious Oliver. "You know what I think about you two, and how it's not right, but it's your business, and he's certainly not mine and never will be".

"Why would she want to make up lies or upset other people just to get at you? It's sick and it's crazy", Lauren's crying; perhaps with relief, or perhaps with the flow of horrible thoughts all jumbling around that I'm all too familiar with. Taking her other hand, I try my best to explain why She would do this and, most likely, with His support. I give her even more detail of what I'd been through with all the same stuff for three years, before running and ending up here.

"It was Hell and, frankly, still is. It's messed me up. The lies, and stalking, and accusations, all wrapped up in this disgusting sexual stuff. It's made me... not right... I can't even begin to tell you how sick in the head I've been... the stuff I've done!" Now I'm crying, and she's stopped walking. Stock still, she's looking at me, unblinking, with her head cocked in interest. I've said too much.

"Fuck. Forget I said anything, please. I just want you to know all this", my hand drawing a circle around my face. "*All this* isn't what it seems. I'm not as normal as you think, and I'm not as strong! But I would never go near Oliver whether he's with you or whether he's not".

"I'm not stupid. I know he likes you a lot, Lola". My heart tugs for her.

"So what?! I don't like him! Not to mention, I think he's a bit of a dick". This makes her laugh, but I know she's in pain. "Let's walk on a bit more, dry our faces off, and pretend it was the sea air that made us look like tomatoes". Tucking her scarf more securely around her neck, and righting her cardigan where it's slipped to expose her tanned shoulders, I give her a little shake.

"Ok then - no more of that rubbish. Let's go", she says and starts to walk ahead of me.

****

"Do you know where my mum is?" reads the message from Sam. "No. Why?" I reply, almost breathless that he's not asking to see me again. "She went out last night and I haven't seen her since. She said she was going out with you". A flicker of unease catches in my chest.

Carolanne and I had agreed to go out to a pub in the next village, but with her moods changing like the weather, and knowing how quick to anger she is with me, I just couldn't handle another drama or crisis... even if it was as small as arguing with a barmaid, or falling in the street!

"I decided not to go out, Sam. I didn't think your mum would go out herself". We're on the phone now and I'm more than a little anxious, so the call felt necessary. She might be hard work these days, but she is my friend and she's got Sam to think about, never mind her tenure at the pub. "I'll try ringing her and see if I can track her down. You do what you can to get the pub ready for when she gets back, or maybe phone someone to take her hours on today. Aye, that's best. Get her work covered, and I'll find her and sort her out, if needs be."

Three hours, 16 calls, five messages and a dozen frantic texts later, Carolanne's voice booms into my ear. "Whaddyawant? I'm having fun!" she slurs. It's worse than I predicted. I've never known her like this.

"Sam's worried, and I'm coming to get you. It's half 11 in the bloody morning!"

"Don't shpeak to me like that, nosey bitch. I'll do what I want. The kid's fine. Leave me alone." My stomach hardens in anger. I'm sick to death of being spoken to like crap and, if I had a son, I wouldn't be disappearing off overnight and not telling him where I was going or who with. The kid (oh god, kid!) has no one else in the world.

"Don't fucking speak to me like that. Where are you? I'm coming to fetch you. You're acting pathetic!" She goes quiet, but I hear heavy breathing and then puffs of air as she sucks noisily on a cigarette. She's with someone, I think, as her preference is roll-ups.

"I'm at Bruce's house. Come join the party", her tone's all friendly and nice now.

Taking the chance and glad of the change of pace in her attitude, I scratch the address down and thank the gods I know where she's ended up. It's actually quite a nice area, further down the coast, about a 20-minute drive away.

An hour later, I'm driving along the coast road with Carolanne singing at the top of her lungs, in a top stained with red wine, and squinty hair bun bobbing in the breeze through the open window. She's a mess, and I don't think it's just alcohol, either. "Take me to the chemist. Need to get the morning after pill, then I'm coming to yours. No way am I going home to take a comedown on my own!"

Carolanne's minor meltdown with some guy called Bruce and copious chemicals did seem to be another ladder-step downwards in our relationship. It was like she hated me seeing her flaws or knowing her mistakes; not that I was one to judge. I barely batted an eyelid, and easily drained the booze out of her system with cup of tea after cup of tea, and hour after hour watching telly in my bed, while I worked downstairs. She stayed for two nights in the end, and I rather liked the company. Over those few days, she was quite warm and nice with me, but the moody, catty, Carolanne returned not long after and, in fact, slightly worse.

"Are you going to get back with Robert?" the message reads. I'm in the bath a few days after the cliff walk with Lauren, and about a week, maybe two, after his mum's night out.

"No, Sam, I'm not. He's a creep and his girlfriend's a nutter". I finish it with a row of laughing emojis. "Well, you can always see me again?" he chances, cheekily followed up with some green hearts and his own selection of laughing emojis. "Told you. Never again. Friends only", I reply.

He doesn't send another message and goes offline quickly. I hate hurting him and putting him off, but the fact is, it should never have happened, once was enough. Banging my fists on the side of the bath hurts, and water splashes the tiles. "Fucking stupid idiot bitch, Lola!" I shout, and not for the first time these last few weeks.

My phone rings but I ignore it. I make myself a drink and choose what to wear. It's a Saturday; a big night in any pub, and Carolanne's is no exception. Now high Summer, the village is in full party-mode. It's been hot every day for months; we're all tanned, but getting itchy for a little rain. There's a beach party and bonfire later, a yearly tradition, apparently, so I choose denim shorts and a white off-the-shoulder top.

Buttoning the shorts and reaching for my phone, I decide to read the message but have no intention of replying to Sam again. This has to stop. Three times he's asked to repeat the mistake, and three's a crowd, as I well know.

"We should have a threesome, baby", He said once after we got back together again. Aghast, I'd denied him immediately, only to find out he'd been watching porn of the same nature, and masturbating, while I got dressed for my birthday dinner. "It's your fault, anyway. If you gave me what I wanted, I wouldn't need that stuff. All guys do it. Even at work we watch it during shift-breaks", he'd said calmly, then walked away down the hall as I cried in the shower, desperately trying to wash away what I'd seen, and how cruel he was.

Feeling sick and dirty all over again reminds me, the leaflet that Kay gave me for those meetings; I don't think I even took it out of my pocket. Phoebe looks up with interest, expecting me to reach for her lead next to my jacket, and then rests her head in disappointment when I shake my own. "Not just now, Pheebs – mummy needs to fix her head better". Checking who called, I see it was a withheld number, no message. "Sales most likely", I whisper, but feeling that thud of dread between my eyes.

Pouring a drink and smoothing the leaflet to iron out the creases, I sit and put my feet up on the window ledge, and take a sip. "Talking for Recovery", the leaflet reads. "A group of people who believe that sharing our dark sides makes our lives lighter" I'm not sure about that; a bit too close to home for me, I think. Mind you, I'd try anything to get better. Feel better. Be a better person.

I say the last sentence out loud, and Phoebe wags her tail. "Yep. I'll give it a go!" She stands up and walks across the room to me Staffy-Smiling. "Remind me to speak to Kay at the thing later". Phoebe wags her tail so hard that her entire body moves and, with a plan of action at hand, I let myself smile.

"Do you want a drink?" Oliver's standing over me, backlit by the bonfire so huge, it looks like a giant made it.

"No - I'm fine, thanks", I reply as politely, yet pointedly, as I can manage.

"Oh, come on - don't be like that!" he says, sitting down heavily next to me. "I know you don't like me, and it's my fault for coming on strong when I first met you . I was just totally blown away when you arrived, and I made a mess of it". He's still talking but I wish he wouldn't.

My heart flickers as I catch Lauren's eye; she's a few metres away talking to Kay, Carolanne and someone I recognise from one of the local shops. "Let me get you a drink to say sorry". Before I can say no again, he's up and walking away barefooted across the sand, to the small makeshift bar.

"Fuck!" I hiss under my breath, and consider walking away.

"What did he say?" Lauren's suddenly beside me, hands on hips, and furious. Her eyes are lit by the flames and red from rage, not fire.

"Nothing. He apologised for being a knob when we first met. I told you about that on the Cliffs the other week". I wish he hadn't fucking come anywhere near me, now she's all rattled again. Last thing I need is another one of my so-called friends being difficult. Carolanne's hard work enough and, right now, the less drama I have, the more chance I have of getting myself sorted out, maybe even sobered up; now that would be a good idea, seeing the horrendous choices I've made when blasted!

Oliver's walking back towards us, a wide smile on his face and holding two drinks, not three. Lauren notices this at the same time I do, and shoots me a look of hate. "Oliver got you a drink, Lauren; I told him I didn't want one, so that's yours", I say loudly as he approaches. His step falters, and I see by the way he changes his smile that he clicks.

"Yeah, babe, that's your one", he pushes it into her hand and walks away, towards Carolanne and the others.

"He's pissing me off, and maybe you shouldn't wear such revealing clothes, Lola!" she says, but doesn't wait for a reply. She's gone and I'm left alone.

Thinking about going home, I'm walking along the shore, listening to everyone but me having a good time. Maybe this is what I deserve; the gods are punishing me for what I did. Karma's creeping and nipping at my heels, and the little life I've tried to build away from Her and Him has started crumbling, rotting away. I've betrayed my one of my friends in the worst of ways, by sleeping with her son. I've hurt his heart, maybe broken it, by refusing his advances. And now my best friend, the one I trust most here in Bridgefell, is riddled with insecurity and thinks I'm cheating, or at least going to cheat, with the man she's adored for a decade.

Facing the sea, I finish my drink and make the decision to go home. Turning, I walk straight into Kay again. Laughing at how we keep doing this, she turns me to look at the see again. "You obviously have stuff going on up in there", she says, lightly tapping my forehead.

"You could say that", I mutter loud enough for her to hear.

"Have you given any more thought about coming to the meetings with me? There's one next week. I'll drive as I think you might need a drink after it". Shame burns my face; she knows I drink too much; I think everyone knows, they just don't know why or care enough to even come close to understanding.

"One meeting won't hurt. All we do is talk and share the stuff that makes us feel bogged down. Sometimes folk offer advice, sometimes we don't need it. It's private and no one else from Bridgefell goes, so you don't need to worry about that". She's determined, I'll give her that.

"You should be in sales, Kay", I say, bending to lift my silver sandals off the sand. The sunset lights up the battered, peeling, leather as though they are covered in sequins, bringing them back to new.

"I was, once", she replies, and the tone of her voice makes me stand up abruptly. "That's for another time. Come to the meeting. I think you'll be surprised at the secrets people have and how it helps to share."

"Go on, then. Not much to lose, have I?!" I start to turn.

"Don't be daft! Folk like you, Lola, and you have blokes all over the shop chasing you. It's just taking a bit of time to settle in, now you're starting to spot the sleazes!" She takes my arm, and we walk back to the party.

Carolanne watches us as we walk towards the group where she's loudly holding court. "Here they are! Besties forever!" She shouts aggressively, and is grinning like a tiger. She's drunk; I recognise that tone and realise she's angry again, too. Resisting the urge to snap at her, I put my shoes on and declare my intention to go home, lying about an early morning shift at the deli . "Scaredy cat!" she yells after me, but I don't turn around.

She's getting nastier with me every day. Come to think of it, she started getting dark with me after I stood up to her over Sam's room, but things definitely worsened after she stayed with me, sobering up. Unsure what this means or how to handle it and, frankly, too tired to think straight, I head to the little bus stop near the beach. The last bus is due and so, as I tipsily trip a little up the Jacobs Ladder steps from the beach, is my bed.

Listen to: Tina Turner – River Deep, Mountain High

Chapter 10: Perfect

August arrived, announcing herself all red ribbons and firework sunsets. I'd forgotten what rain felt like. Looking at the dried out and drooping hedgerows that, in January, had been proud and tall, I'm almost sad for them now. Feeling tired and dried out myself, I'd agreed to go to the meeting with Kay, and felt genuine hope that it may in some way help ease the shame and guilt that were bubbling and boiling my brain all of the time.

The vicious cycle of anxiety-triggering risk-taking behaviours had, in the past, been so low-level it was barely visible. Stealing a little red pencil when I was eight, skiving off school and hiding in the garden shed when I was 11, even kissing the wrong boy who already had a girlfriend when I was 18; even letting Jamie steal me away from my Husband. All those together were nothing compared to the fact that I'd never, ever, broken such a huge moral rule or law! Thing is, the anxiety only ever got worse and this time, the feelings of paranoia and fear are raw and wide-ranging and terrible and vast.

"You look skinny again. What's up with you?" Kay's asking, as she starts the engine and backs out of the car park.

"Nothing. Just working too hard and not sleeping enough. Funny phone calls, too". This is the first time I've acknowledged out loud that the calls are troubling me.

"What do you mean funny, phone calls?" Kay slides her sunglasses on and speeds up out of the village, still carefully watching the road for any careless, hungover, tourist eagerly looking for somewhere to satisfy a thirst.

Letting out a long sigh, I rub my eyes and rest the side of my head on the cool of the car window. "It's not the first time. When I was with Him, She used to call and text and use fake accounts, or get her mates to do it. Other times, it was females He was cheating on me with. But those times, most of them, I'd get abuse, names, threats that sort of thing".

Kay glances sharply at me, but quickly looks back at the road. She licks her lips and I feel a prickle of unease. "And can you hear anyone in these calls? Anything at all?" she asks. These are the sorts of questions the police used to ask; she seems... experienced.

"Well, at first it was just breathing, and I think I heard a lighter, like the person was lighting a cigarette; but I'm so tired and stressed out, I could have imagined it. My head's all over the place. I don't think I can do this again". Tears fill my eyes as I choke back a sob.

Kay puts her hand on my leg. "Well, put a call recorder app thing on your phone, and then I can listen with you next time it happens".

"How do you know about all this stuff?" Leaning forward, I reach for a tissue off the dashboard.

"My husband was a police officer. He did a lot of stalking cases... before we split up," she says, not looking at me.

Sensing it best not to ask more about this, I blow my nose and try not to cry as I explain a little more why I came to find myself in Bridgefell, eight months ago.

"That's horrendous, what happened to you. No wonder you look like a little broken bird," she says, stopping the car outside a community centre that I'd only ever driven past. The lights are on inside and, out of nowhere, I feel absolutely terrified. I shouldn't be here, whatever these meetings are about, or whoever comes to them - they aren't like me. They are just normal people who've made silly mistakes. I'm not normal and neither's my mistake.

"I think maybe this isn't for me, Kay. I'll go for a walk along there, around the park and get a coffee. Meet you back here in an hour." I'm backing away but she has my hand tight in hers.

"Stop being a wimp. It's not some sort of cult, and no one's being sacrificed. Well, not tonight, anyway!" She smiles a crooked smile, and looks genuinely concerned that I'm not going in with her.

Maybe she told them I was coming. I don't want to embarrass her. Fuck. "Ok. But I don't think I'm going to talk or anything. Just watch and listen, suss things out. If that's ok?" She squeezes my hand and somehow gets me through the double doors into bright light, and where the smell of coffee and cake greets me.

There is a circle of about a dozen wooden chairs in the far corner of the room, which is as standard as any 1970's community hall can get. A shiny but battered wooden floor, a stage for a play or concert at one end, and a makeshift kitchenette or a bar at the other. The stage is set as though for a play, or a drama class, with a throne at centre-stage, perhaps Macbeth or Sleeping Beauty.

Taking all this in, tiny details one at a time, makes me feel a little better; this could be any sort of meeting, for any group, on any topic. It's going to be fine. The room's even unusually warm which I'm glad of; growing up, no matter how warm it was outside, the village hall was always freezing, and the cold has always rattled my nerves and made me jumpy.

"Come on, let's get the hard bit over with!" Kay's lightly tugging me across to a small cluster of people. I count seven, and don't recognise anyone, until Lauren turns to face me. My chest catches alight with fear, she smiles and winks, but doesn't acknowledge me. Friendly enough? The Oliver thing must be forgotten. Thank god for that.

She has been a lot more chilled with me this last week, actually; I think my showing her I wasn't interested on the beach, rather than just saying I wasn't, genuinely helped. Relief has me reaching for a slice of cake! I don't eat cake!

"I made that". A voice over my shoulder. An older man with grey hair and a belly that says he makes and eats a lot of cake, is standing beside me.

"Looks good! I cook but don't have a sweet tooth," speaking through coffee cake crumbs makes him smile. Ok, so far, so good.

"You're very welcome to the group, Lauren," says another voice. Spinning around, I'm greeted by someone even smaller than I am; long dyed black hair, and the look of someone who needs these meetings perhaps more than me.

"I like your hair", is all I can think of to say, she looks so vulnerable; all I can think of are words to that effect. Then I realise, we aren't to use our full names, or share too much of our lives, other than our secrets; No one's making small talk; too easy to slip and breach confidentiality.

"I think that's all of us for tonight. The hot weather's getting on people's nerves and making them want to stay indoors, faces pressed up to fans, drinking cold drinks, and wishing for September". Walking out of the shadows and towards us, I don't recognise the woman, but she's clearly the chair of today's meeting.

Officious and organised, she slides glasses down onto her nose and take us all in, one by one, and make what appear to be ticks on a notepad. She suddenly slaps it shut and puts it under her chair. Thank god she doesn't make notes! It's just an attendance list in case of fire or something. The cake slides back down my throat.

"Who wants to start tonight's meeting, make the first share?" the glasses lady asks. Out of the corner of my eye, I see Lauren's left hand flicker; it doesn't go unmissed by Glasses Lady "Lauren, would you like to start? It's been a while since you shared and, actually, since you came to a meeting. Lovely to have you back, and glad you are ready to forgive yourself again".

It's a little surreal this thing I'm at, the airy-fairy wording and soft lighting. A bit hippyish and almost like AA was, when

I used to go with Jamie, when I thought alcohol was his drug, not other human being's bodies. There's the cake sliding up my throat again. "Well, I've had some bad thoughts recently. Not very nice thoughts. I feel terrible and it's affecting a part of my life that's really important to me. A friendship," Lauren's talking so I snap out of it and listen.

Sipping at the cup of ice-cold water someone's placed in my hand, without me noticing; looking around, I try to work out who might have given it to me, to see if they are looking at me. Kay nods, and I smile gratefully. I'd almost forgotten she was here.

"So. I've had nasty thoughts about a friend and know it's not right and it's made me behave really nastily and I have to make amends for it. The last time this happened, I lost a good friend and was really gutted, to be honest, and I don't want it to happen again". Lauren's looking directly at me.

Rooted to the seat, I know I'm starting to blush, but the rest of the group pretends not to notice. "My boyfriend has what you call a wandering eye, and well... wandering hands... and I put up with it, but he likes to go for my friends. It's his thing. So I thought it was happening again and that she, my friend, had done like the others and given in to him. But I realised recently she hadn't. Another person had been winding me up a bit and I listened to them; it all just got messy and I feel really bad". Lauren's face puffs up and a fat tear falls down her cheek.

I make the smallest movement to go to her but the grey-haired man to my left grabs my knee and shakes his head. I get the message; the rules here are talk about our guilt, not fix it. Not show anyone who we are, and only say what we need to say to lift the clouds of remorse; not help anyone do it for themselves.

"Do you feel better, now you've had a chance to open up about this, Lauren?" the girl with long black hair asks.

"I do. It's not who I am, this angry and jealous thing. I hate feeling this way", Lauren sniffs into her tissue but doesn't look at me this time.

"I think we all get the Green-Eyed Monster every now and again", Kay's speaking this time. "I know when my husband left me for someone else, I was... well, I wasn't in my right mind, to be honest. Those thoughts, wow! Very difficult to live with, never mind suppress". So that's why she's a bit cranky or, at least, watchful of those of us in the friendship group who seem to her, perhaps, to not take relationships seriously enough. Coming here's been useful already, so far! I feel bad for judging Kay when I first met her; she's simply been burned, as so many of us have.

The meeting continues with more shares and exchanges from others in the group; a shoplifter who's thinking about "lifting" again, someone riddled with guilt for not visiting their mother who died the following day, and even the Glasses Lady shared - her guilt for not sharing her inheritance equally between her two children. "I just don't love them the same", she said and a few of the group nodded, more than I expected, to be honest.

Two hours later, Kay and I are saying our goodbyes at the backdoor to the deli. "Are you glad you came even, though you didn't share?" she asks, leaning against her car and folding her arms.

"Yes. I know I'm not supposed to, but I felt like I understood you and Lauren a bit better. Now I have more stuff to share about feeling bad, about maybe misunderstanding you when I first came here!" Kay laughs and lifts herself away from the car.

"Don't worry about that; it's a small place. Close-knit, and no one's perfect". The last word seems to echo around the empty car park as she drives away.

Tossing and turning in bed that night, I couldn't drift off to sleep. Phoebe grumpily lumbered off to her own bed about 3am. That upset me even more, as I hate sleeping without her. "Suit yourself!" I hissed, and she burrowed her face deeper into the blankets. "Might as well go and do some prep downstairs. I can see I'm not wanted here". Huffily, I put a hoody on over my short pyjamas and stomp downstairs, flicking every light on along the way.

My phone buzzes, I'd put it on silent as usual once in bed. "Bitch you're going to get set on fire" the message reads. "I'm going to anally rape you" the next one comes in; whoever's sending these is online on Facebook now, live. I almost fall down the last few steps. Breathless, dizzy and afraid, I reply "Who is this? Another one of Jamie's sluts again?" The message is read but then they go offline and block me.

It's just like last time. How've they found me? My Facebook's a different name and there's no way He could have guessed Cornwall, and She's sneaky but not that smart. Shaking with shock, I make a coffee and pour in a generous amount of brandy .

"Here we go again", I whisper, drinking it back in one.

Listen to: Nididi O – No Mercy

Chapter 11: A Woman Scorned

Pulling back from Carolanne has been easier than I expected; she was never that good at playing "besties" anyway, even at the start. Equality, friendship... softness, were never going to be words I'd use to describe her friendship ethos! But I liked her confidence, her way of working a room and, at one time, I felt safe in her power. Like I wanted her to be in control and telling me what to do.

In a strange way, I felt mothered then, not smothered but the opposite; neglected, with spikes of something I couldn't quite put my finger. Like searching for a pulse, I never found a sense of true safety in being around her, no matter how hard I looked, or how gently I pressed. I was vulnerable when we met, and had a very warped view on how friendships worked. To me, she was Jamie. Now, she still is, but has all Jamie's bad qualities now.

The Sam thing wasn't even the trigger point for my ending the friendship with Carolanne; it was the setup with Robert, and then the growing flood of nasty comments, dark looks, and unreasonable demands that I jump to her aid whenever she felt like it. Only yesterday, she demanded I "come now, do a French plait" on her hair, for some last-minute meeting with some new guy. I hated myself, scurrying across the road, not even washed, and dressed for the day, hoping no one would see me, but hoping even more she'd be in a good mood for a change.

"Hurry up! He's collecting me soon!" she yelled from the top of the stairs as I rushed through the back door. Disappearing from view, she gave me an opportunity to stop, take a deep breath, and hold back the reaction she deserved: "Don't speak to me like that or I won't plait anything!"

Instead, I ran up the stairs, already sweating, hoping she knew where the hairbrush was or I'd be searching for it, while she shadowed me, muttering and swearing about me being stupid.

Once I started quietly plaiting, I noticed my hands trembling, not from last night's over-indulgences, but from fear. Fear of her. Tying the end neatly with a hair-bobble, I knew then; it was time to tie up the loose ends of this toxic friendship. There was no way I was doing it to her face! God, no! Fragile and anxious enough, I knew it was best to gently pull back and, if she pushed, just say I felt things had run their course and it was best we didn't spend so much time together.

Of course, the final nail in the coffin came quickly; almost as though she knew I was for the off.

* * * * * * * * * * * * * *

"Why are you blanking me?" She's staring me straight on, leaning over the bar, right in my personal space.

"I'm not. Just busy with Jen's place and I have my own stuff going on. That's all", I can't make eye contact and she knows it. I've never been one for confrontations on the passive aggressive or awkward scale. Bring me a full-on fight, make me angry, then yes; we have a battle. But needle me slowly, quietly, and try to make me feel uncomfortable, and I'm neither use nor ornament.

"Typical of you: sneaky and selfish", she says and, without waiting for my reply, spins away, turns a big smile on and starts serving a regular further down the bar. Feeling her eyes on my back as I head outside, there's an inescapable feeling of impending doom cloaking my shoulders and tightening around my neck.

"You were warned", Lauren said as I described the encounter.

"I know. I just wanted to fit in, and she was nice in the beginning and now I feel trapped and it's a bloody mess. It's a small place and she's a big personality. Should never have got caught up in her orbit!" replying quietly, so Carolanne doesn't overhear, even if she's hiding in the shadows of the doorway. I know I'm paranoid as all hell and deserve it. I've gone from one abusive relationship to another. Seamlessly.

My phone starts to ring so, sliding it across the table, I turn it screen up. "Private number again?" Lauren's taking the phone and clicking the red phone to end the call.

"Yeah. It's Natalie, or maybe Sharna or Jamie. It'll stop soon, it always does. I've more to worry about than those two idiots and their bonkers games".

"You've a nice collection of nutters there! I'm going to start calling you Stupid Squirrel! Gathering nuts like nobody's business! So yes, good plan. Let's go and get something to eat", Lauren's chuckling at her joke and pushing her chair back. I watch her slipping her cardigan off the back of it. I'm glad she doesn't want to talk more about it; it's exhausting trying to work out why people behave like this and how to deal with it, all over again.

My head hurts from last night and there's a ringing in my ears that started up a few days ago. It comes first thing in the morning once the day starts and the night-terrors stop. It's like the images and fears won't let me go, even during the day.

"Don't fucking come near this place again!" Carolanne's text comes in as soon as we cross the road. Turning around, I see movement as she slides fast away from the doorway back to the shadows, where I am beginning to think she belongs. Oddly, I'm not surprised at the texts that come next. "Fucking tramp", the next message arrives by the time Lauren and I reach the door to my flat.

Throughout that night in early August, the heat of Carolanne's rage is worse than I expected. Numbness and relief that we weren't going to fake the friendship anymore slid into panic and dread, when I realised she was, potentially, just as psycho as Jamie and Sharna. Maybe even worse. At least Sharna was a covert psycho: all lies, fake accounts, and sneaking around destroying my life. Carolanne is now showing all the signs of an overt psycho, a type I'd never before experienced.

****

The black paint bleeds all the way from the top of the door down to the steps leading up to my flat. No, it's actually been thrown so hard, there's splashback and it's streaked the stone steps; it's even been thrown over a series of bikes for hire and a plant pot at the bottom of the steps. There's a smell of gas so strong I panic for a second, thinking she's waiting inside ready to set fire to the deli kitchen . Then I realise it's the smell of the paint.

It's been several weeks since Carolanne and I "parted ways", but she doesn't seem to realise that ending a friendship means just that, an actual ending. Instead, she's started this one-sided war. A war I have no interest in tooling up for and wading into, not since what happened with Jamie and Sharna. Nope! Not... A... Chance!

I've started going to The Forgivers Club meetings each week; anything to have space to breathe and talk without judgement or advice. No one can help me, and I don't expect anyone to either. It's purely a swap of poison in my head for oxygen, even if it's only for 60 blessed minutes. Naming no names is easy; I can't even bring myself to mention Carolanne. Her behaviour's mirroring both Jamie and Sharna's at home, and has ignited a deep, dark depression that I'm slowly sinking deeper and deeper into. Sadly, when I am victimised and isolated, I get angry, reckless and... dangerous.

Only last night, Carolanne ranted and raved about how old and fat I was, and how I had "no home and no friends" on WhatsApp. Naïve to how bold and brave she'd be, I didn't expect such a tirade alongside her very own profile picture, with even her number boldly on show. I knew, then, that it was time to involve the police.

What little I do know about sociopaths is that they fear no one and nothing, and have no boundaries. That, for me, could be very, very dangerous. She was right on one thing, though; I did indeed have no home and no one, bar my fragile friendship with Lauren, complex reliance on Kay, and my beloved dog.

"Nothing and no one" rang around and around and around for days before I plucked up the courage to make the call. A call that became the first of many.

* * * * * * * * * * * * *

"We'll go and see her. Have a word. See what happens from there", the police officer's rocking back and forth on his heels. It's making me nauseous, like being on a boat alongside him.

"Is that all you can do? Really?!" Shock and familiarity, of yet another situation where I'm powerless, are making my breaths come too fast; a panic attack is on the way.

"Well, getting evidence from these online site things…" he pokes at my phone, like it's a smelly shoe, "… are notoriously difficult, Miss Hague". The officer, a something-or-other Trevenna, starts to step back towards my door, where you can still see the remnants of the paint attack of last month. The silver doorknob has slashes of black paint from Carolanne's frantic hurling, and even the fresh, navy blue paint I used on the door itself still smells new.

"But it's been weeks! Nearly two months! I've shown you all sorts and look! *Look!* The WhatsApp account the messages came from even has her picture and her number!" Openly crying, and doing a full-blown Crazy Lady routine, make Phoebe scuttle from between my legs, away to her bed in the other room. "This isn't right! You can't just leave me to it! *Surely?!*"

Trevenna is unsympathetic and rather cold. "She'll get bored and leave you alone soon, I'm sure", are the last words I hear, as he practically runs down the steps away from me.

Speechless and confused, I sit on the step with the messages glaring at me, and cry; and not for the first time today. "If this is how she is just because we aren't friends anymore, what the hell will she be like if she ever finds out about what happened with Sam?!" I wail as Phoebe, pressed up against me, starts to shake.

This is all too familiar to her, as well; we came here for friendship and peace, and I've fucked it up in all colours of the rainbow in less than a year. I've been here nine months and it feels like I have, indeed, given birth to The Devil.

Ruffling Phoebe's fur, the tears squeeze my throat again, but I look up instinctively, just as the bus to the next village wheels its way into the bus stop across the road. The sudden thought of getting out of here, even for an afternoon, feels like a miracle just happened.

Refilling Phoebe's water bowl, and tipping food into her dish, I know I have at least five minutes before it turns and then waits at the other bus stop for the return trip along the coast, stopping at a pub I've been to a few times since Carolanne and I fell out. I don't know if it's even a "fall out", but what else is it? She knows nothing of my terrible secret and yet this, to anyone else, is simply two women arguing! Even though I haven't retaliated, yet.

Grabbing my beach bag, purse, and sunglasses, I leave the flat and as I turn to lock the door, I can see through the little window, and watch Phoebe plop down onto her bed and nestle her nose into the blankets. My heart squeezes, but I take a deep breath and start jogging down the stairs, fixated on the doors of the bus. "Stay strong, Lola. Stay strong", I whisper. Distracted, I don't see who's also approaching the bus.

"Fucking bitch!" The shouting behind me signals Carolanne. That deep, husky, angry, voice is unmistakeable. Wherever I go, she's there. Whatever I do, she knows it.

Running faster and jumping onto the bus, I see my neighbour smoking on his front step; he's seen her, too. Now, surely now, the police can do something properly? *A witness!* That's the first time piece of good luck I've had in a long time. Setting an alarm to remind me to call the police with this the next morning, I breathe a small sigh of relief. Opening the window on the seat opposite me, the breeze catches my hot face and I close my eyes in what may, actually, be relief. I just want her to stop and leave me alone. That's all.

"She looks nuts!" a voice shouts from the front; it's the driver. "She always was a wild one! What'd you do?!" He laughs but I don't even smile.

"As far as she knows, all I've done is not be friends anymore".

"Hell hath no fury!" he yells over his shoulder at me. "You're not the first and you won't be the last! But if I were you, keep your head down and don't go near her again". Helpful advice if this was a normal situation! I have nowhere else to go and even if I did run, I don't have the energy to start over, not just now anyway. I have a terrible feeling that Carolanne is just getting started. I wonder what the driver means by, "You're not the first"?

Too tired, and afraid of his answer, I don't ask and shut the conversation down. "Thanks for the advice!" I shout back over the revving of the engine as we go up the hill and leave the village behind.

"Can I get you a drink?" Curly-ish light brown hair and, I think, hazel eyes; he's no super-model, but he's ok, I guess. If I were more drunk, he could be my type although I prefer them taller.

"Go on then. I'll be over there, it's my turn for pool". He grins widely and I feel him watching me as I walk away, choose a cue, and squat at the table, ready to start the game with my last 50 pence piece. I've been here nearly two hours and, to be honest, I'm tired. I think the bus back to the village is in 10 minutes.

"Are you good then?" He's back, but his body is a little too close. I can't put my finger on it but he's familiar, although I'm sure I've never met him. "My name's Steph and you can call me Steph". Grinning at his joke and handing me my drink, he doesn't break eye contact.

"Sure", I reply, not giving him my name. I feel uneasy, and take a shot to break the balls on the table. If I were feeling more alive, I could break his balls. No problem.

"Want to go somewhere after this? After you win?" he's back, close to me again and his hand brushes my hip. Warning bells ring aloud now. The name Steph and his over-familiar way....

"No. It's ok. I'm ready for home. Work tomorrow", I reply, neatly potting a ball. I've gone off him fast, and I think he knows it.

"Come on. I'll take you to that posh place up on the hill. My treat", he presses. Now I'm definitely off him. The place he's talking about sits alone, a manor house in large grounds, is accessible only by car or a by a long walk on a secluded hillside path. The alarm bells ring louder.

"Really, I'm fine, thanks. Been there, food was rubbish", I want him away from me, but I don't know why.

"Fuck you then, bitch", he hisses in my ear. Then I know who he is. He's a friend of Carolanne's. She's mentioned a Steph once or twice; I think I saw his picture once. Back when we were friends, she showed off all the guys she'd been with. It took over an hour and that was just her Facebook.

He's gone like a rabbit from foxes. Straight through the crowd. All I see is the back of his jacket, and then the people he's pushed through come back together again, totally oblivious to what just happened. Carolanne knew where I was going when she chased me towards the bus. Maybe she even followed in her car?! She's had time to contact him, arrange for him to come here, to try and lure me somewhere, alone, and private. *Jesus Christ!* This is beyond anything I could have imagined. I need to leave this place; not just the pub, but Bridgefell. Get away, far, far away.

"This is going to be my last meeting. I've been offered a job in Newcastle". The lie comes easily, even though I'm amongst The Forgivers. " I leave in the next few weeks. If I leave it longer than that, the job goes to someone else". Looking at my knees, I see goosebumps appear like a rash. It's early October, and colder than I expected.

The Summer treated us too well, and now our punishment is an extra-chilly Autumn breeze that doesn't seem to stop whipping off the sea, catching me by surprise whenever I venture out.

"Oh! Well, that's a surprise! We thought you liked it here!" Cake Man is visibly upset.

"I did. I do. It's just time to move on. The bit of trouble I've mentioned a few times just isn't calming down; in fact, it's getting worse". The goosebumps get bigger.

I'm terrified Sam will tell his mother what happened, especially when he hears I'm leaving. For all I know, he has his mother's vindictive streak, not that I wouldn't deserve it from him. I hurt him, badly.

We share a small wave across the street or sad smile in the local shop, but we haven't had contact since my last "no" to meeting up again. It feels a lifetime ago, but it's only two months, maybe less. I don't know, I try not to think about it. Deep in denial, I'm just about managing to breathe in and out, with Carolanne's harassment and my fear of Jamie and Sharna making an appearance here in the village. My small piece of Heaven has turned too fast into Hell, and it's all my fault.

"Don't get upset! These things happen! Women are always the worst when it comes to fall outs!" Glasses Lady has crossed the circle of chairs and is kneeling in front of me; she's cupping my face in her warm, papery, hands.

"You have no idea how I've messed up. It's all my fault!" Something inside me shatters. I can't live like this anymore.

The calls, the messages. The gossip and lies! I don't think I leave the house more than once a week, and that's just to run to the shop if a delivery for the deli is missing an item or two. I think she's going to kill me". The words tumble over each other and the room falls deathly silent.

The flush of relief at letting the fear explode and fill the room has me prattling on and on and on, not caring what they might think; I just want forgiveness, to run and escape, and never look back.

It must have been only two or three minutes but my whole insides are empty and numb with tiredness and lack of holding it all in; I sit there hunched over in my chair sobbing. The sounds echo and it takes only a few beats for me to realise that the usual squeaking of chairs as The Forgivers nod in support and murmurs of sympathy are not chasing my own voice around the room.

Looking up, I see Lauren in the doorway, slightly in shadow because of the autumn light and today's later-than-normal meeting. All eyes aren't on me now, they're on her. "You didn't. Lola... tell me you didn't!" she whispers but we all hear her.

It's a badly kept secret that she and I are close friends, and an even worse-kept secret that we're from the same village. The same village a well-known mad woman lives with her recently-turned 16-year-old son. Comfortable in this place, we'd let things slip, and felt secure in the strict confidentiality values of the group. It's been a mistake.

The door slams and I hear her car start up. Still no one speaks. Then Cake Man does. "You'd better go. Yes, best you go. Now". He looks unfamiliar now; angry, an odd shade of grey mottled pink. Infected with my shame he knows we've shared here for weeks, and I'm a monster.

"Go!" Glasses Lady says, standing up so fast her chair falls over.

The sound shakes me out of my own chair and I'm running, running, and running. Running past my car, running down to the pebbled shore. Stumbling and sobbing, slipping and falling. I fall and get up several times before running into the waves, struggling to stay on my feet, crying and shouting that I'm sorry, over and over, until Kay pulls me back to the shore.

I can't stop shouting that I'm sorry, and she clamps her hand over my mouth. "Shut up!" she shouts then repeats it, quieter.

Sand fills my mouth and saltwater goes up my nose. "I'm sorry! I'm sorry! It's my fault. I know that! I just want to leave! Get away from her, him, her, them, all of it!"

"Shut up, I said". She throws herself on the sand next to me, and pushes me to a sitting position. "Look. Just fucking get a grip, Lola. This is your fuck-up and you need to face it". She's grinding her teeth and is furious, but not disgusted.

" I know. I know. I don't know how to!" My teeth are chattering, and I start to cough up sand and water.

"Carolanne is a complete psycho. I've known it for years. She targeted me once, a long time ago. It was her who told me about my husband, and she loved every second of it. I felt it. She's not well".

"What do I do, then?" It's pathetic but I'd give anything for someone to tell me.

"You get packed up. You leave. You don't look back. I've seen her in action a few times over the years. She'll stop at nothing to pretty much kill you, or get you to kill yourself first". Kay's voice is flat now, and it's more terrifying than her shouting, and even more frightening than the thought of walking back into that cold, black, sea.

"Get yourself home and take my advice". Kay's standing up, brushing sand off her legs and has her hand out to pull me up beside her. Taking it firmly, I can't help but pull her into my space and squeeze her tight.

"Thank you", I whisper into her hair.

"Look, I've heard of people doing a lot worse, Lola, and you can forgive yourself. What you went through before you came here will have messed you up good and proper. You were looking for comfort and control, and Sam gave you it. You didn't take it! Don't tell another soul what you did. More importantly, don't tell anyone what I just said".

Listen to: AC/DC – Highway To Hell

Chapter 12: Trapped

It's 5am and three days later and I haven't packed a thing. Not that I had much to pack anyway. Pressed close to Phoebe in her bed in the corner, I've just sat and stared at the wall; breaking this position to go to the toilet, and to let Phoebe out for a quick comfort walk. I've been waiting for Carolanne. Every slight noise outside. Every dark flash breaking up the streetlight's beam outside. Every hum of wind through the letterbox. It *all* has me on high alert.

I don't know why I'm not up and gone yet. Maybe I should just face her, get it over with. The look on Lauren's face keeps going over and over, around and around in my head. Phoebe's fur's sticking up like she's waiting for all hell to break loose, too. "I don't want to run anymore. I'm too tired", I whisper, looking up at the wall and half-expecting to see sky and not plasterboard, stained with damp.

"I'm going nuts trapped here", I say, and Phoebe stands up stretching exaggeratedly. She has the right idea. "It's weird that she hasn't come for me yet". Phoebe shakes herself and steps out of her bed to trot over to sit by the door to the fire escape. "Maybe they won't say anything. Keep my secret. It's supposed to be a place for sharing and forgiving, after all." Phoebe wags her tail, and I almost smile.

There's a flicker of hope; Lauren has been a good friend to me, and she won't want Carolanne on the rampage any more than anyone else will. Kay's as afraid of her tirades and punishments as the rest of us. They wouldn't gain anything from telling her what I did. There it is again, a tiny light of hope. "People aren't that cruel. No one could be that cruel!"

My knees creak as I stand properly for the first time all night. Stretching and checking how rough I look in the full-length mirror by the door, Phoebe runs around my legs, full circle, and lets out a small yip of encouragement. Peeking through the fine linen curtain on the window to the street, I wince; there's a weak autumn sun but it's not cold. "Go on then. Let's try a quick walk on the beach. It's early. No one's up yet".

I realise that I'm staggering and my legs are tingling with adrenalin, I walk carefully down to the beach. I've been scared and stressed before, but never felt it physically like this. My heart is fluttering, and nausea overwhelms me. I've heard of people who are mentally ill with stress saying you feel like you are dying, and they are right. I'm scared that my body has gone through *too much*.

Sitting heavily down on the sand, I see stars and my ears start ringing. Phoebe starts to whine, and I blindly reach out to hold her collar, so she's close to me.

"Hey!" His familiar voice makes my chest thud and I almost fall backwards in shock. My mouth fills with bile, and I wipe my mouth on my sleeve; I get up, slowly.

"Sam. You can't be seen talking to me. Walk on. Walk away!" I hiss.

Backing away from him towards the sea, I wrap my scarf tighter and pull my hat down further over my face. Flicking a look left then right, I half expect to see the entire Forgivers Club there, circling us and pointing; chanting "Whore" over and over and over.

"What's up with you?!" He laughs and steps forward to take Phoebe's lead where it's hanging around my neck. Flinching, I step away from him again and pull the lead hard. The clasp on the end catches my ear and it makes me wince in pain, and then the tears come.

"Your mum is stalking me. She won't leave me alone, Sam!" I start crying, and Sam frowns, confused.

"My mum wouldn't do that. She's nuts but she wouldn't do that. Besides, she doesn't know anything. She's her usual bad-tempered shouty self, but she's not said anything. Mind you, I heard her saying to a customer the other day that you fell out and you gave as good as you got!"

"That's a lie! I've said and done nothing! She's relentless, Sam!"

"Oh well. She'll calm down. So you need to calm down!" He's still relaxed and starts to laugh. I have to admit, it's calming me, slowly.

"But they know! At the group thing. It's not even them I'm worried about! It's Lauren. She was so shocked!" Wiping my face on my sleeve again, I look around to make sure no one else is on the beach .

"I don't know her very well, but I do know she can be dramatic. Besides, she's obsessed with Oliver and no one else. She was in the pub last night, all over him. Actually, she was drunk. Very!" Sam's looking out to sea and easily ruffling Phoebe's extra fur beneath her collar. She rolls over in the sand for him to rub her belly, and he laughs again. I'm dumbstruck at how relaxed he is about this. Maybe I should calm myself too. "I'm sorry you're frightened. You didn't do anything wrong. It was my choice, Lola".

He's looking at me, and the rising sun's catching the slightly fluffy facial hair he has on his upper lip, and I start to cry again. "It should never have happened. I took advantage of your feelings to make myself feel better, or maybe feel nothing. It was wrong and I was wrong. I'm not well!"

"Well, it's done now and I'm not sorry", he stands up abruptly. Phoebe spins back around to stand up, eager to go where he's going.

"Sam, I really am sorry", I manage to say before he picks up a stick of seaweed and hurls it into the sea. I watch as Phoebe runs madly after it, her ample rump bobbing and then disappearing into the sea foam. Turning to share a smile with Sam, I'm met with an empty space. He's gone.

****

After our conversation on the beach, I felt better and a little less afraid. Sam's confidence and sense of peace, although sad, was a huge help. I started to venture out of the flat a little more and more each day. I knew it was only a matter of time until Lauren either got in touch, or we bumped into each other, and I'd rehearsed what to say a hundred times before that meeting inevitably happened.

Listen to: Sabrina Carpenter – Lie For Love

Chapter 13: Beaten Down

The shopping's heavier than I expected and Phoebe's trotting a little too far ahead for comfort. "Too bloody confident, that dog" I mutter angrily, and feel beads of sweat prickle under my shirt. "Phoebe! Stop. Wait!" Shouting at her and struggling with the bags, I don't hear the footsteps behind me, but I do feel the dull thud of a fist to the back of my neck.

Turning fast and dropping one of the bags in the process, it takes a few seconds for me to realise someone just punched me. It's Carolanne and she's puce with rage. "Prostitute!" She yells in my face. That's a new one. For the last few months, it's been repeated messages of "Slag", "Tramp" and "Cow", and a few yells if she sees me walking past the pub car park, or if I have the door to the deli open so she can yell inside.

To be honest, I've gotten used to it. She has no idea about Sam and I and, to be fair, I feel so guilty about it that I'm letting her vent her spleen, safe in the knowledge she's only doing it because she can, and not expecting actual physical violence; I've simply been more careful where I go alone, and when I venture out of the flat or bistro in the busier times of the day.

She's basically stalked and harassed me for nearly two months' now. All because I ended the friendship. Numb to the abuse, and glad my secret is safe, I've called and reported every incident, and kept myself to myself wherever possible. "She'll stop soon. Choose someone else", the man who runs the small garage shop said, only last week, when Carolanne drove past and screamed abuse out of the window, *yet again*.

****

"That's what everyone else says. Even the police", I sigh, taking my change from him.

"Do you know why she's doing it? It's madness!" he continues, eager for some gossip. My mouth filled with the words I can't even say: "It's because I slept with her son! She still doesn't know!" I close my eyes tightly and step away from the counter, almost as though the proximity of the kind old man has a truth serum effect.

"She started the night I told her I didn't want to be friends anymore, and basically hasn't stopped. I'm beginning to think she's gay!" the laugh's brittle, but it's a juicy enough theory for Brian, the shopkeeper, to make an "oooooohhhh" sound and step away, to tidy the already pristine shelves. I can see by his neck that he's pink and excited at this possible news.

"So the police aren't doing anything at all?" Brian asks over his shoulder.

"Nope! It's weird as all anything! I can't make sense of it. So far, I haven't had any witnesses which they seem to rely on; but I have lots of evidence and she seems so good at getting me on my own, that I have the suspicion she's either watching me in some way, or has done this to someone else before…"

Brian walks back to the counter and puts his hands on his hips. The camp movement makes me smile, but with tears in my eyes. I falter, and he frowns. "Lola, just keep recording and reporting everything that happens and everything she does". He lays a papery hand on mine, and leans closer. "One day, one time, she will slip up. If she's as angry as you say, and I saw a bit of her rage just now when she drove past, she will make a mistake. And that mistake will create witnesses".

Then the tears do fall, because I am losing hope day by day.

* * * * * * * * * * * * *

It's late afternoon and I am shutting up the deli. Moving from the kitchen at the back of the shop through the small eatery, I'm distracted so I don't see her at the glass door until it's too late.

There's a shattering sound as she kicks the glass. She looks shocked to have been seen, and then runs away. The shop door has had the glass shattered, six times now.

Initially I thought kids, then whoever was making the calls, and now I realise it's been her all along.

Swinging the door frame open, and getting little shards of glass on my shoes, I lean out and shout at her retreating back, "Look, Carolanne. Just let it go! Leave me alone!"

She just speeds up and, within half a minute, disappears inside the pub and slams the door. My eyes catch a movement at an upstairs window, and I think I see Sam disappear behind the partially-closed curtain of the room I know to be Carolanne's living area.

I start sweeping up the glass, and thinking about how to break this news to Jen and Louise. Jen will be upset and shocked, but Louise's default setting is blaming me.

It's a few days later and, having barely left my little flat or the workplace downstairs, I have had peace. It's not good enough, though, as I am fast realising that Carolanne is determined to either isolate me completely, or make me so ill that I do indeed kill myself. I've had to get other people to walk Phoebe, which is up there on the broken heart scale; I'd say an 11 out of 10.

I'm still getting nasty messages and silent phone calls, but I believe these are from Jamie or Sharna, as Carolanne is so vocal; I don't think she would be able to hold in her spite and foul language if she managed to get my new number from Lauren or Kay.

Standing at the window of my bedroom, I peer out from the bottom of the lowered blinds and see a deserted street. It's not yet 9am and the pub is, as usual, dark and closed up. If I take Phoebe for a run on the beach now, I'll have a better chance of avoiding Carolanne.

A spurt of anger at how unfair and cruel this situation is has me reaching for Phoebe's little coat and lead. "Let's go out, baby", I whisper, putting my own coat on. She perks up immediately. "That cunt isn't ruining my life anymore. Or yours, for that matter!" Louder now, this makes my pup stands up, stretch, and wag her tail the hardest I have seen in the last few weeks.

Trotting down the back stairs, out onto the street, a light drizzle starts to fall, but it's not cold and is actually rather pleasant. Not quite smiling, but feeling something like pleasure at the fresh air, I bend down to take Phoebe's lead off; I stand on the pavement to roll my shoulders and do a light stretch ready for a run. I don't see Carolanne running across the street towards me.

Thud. She punches me on the back of the head this time. Harder, but I don't react. It's what she wants.

Half-turning, because I prefer a thump to the back rather than to my face, I step back and start shouting; I'm retaliating in the most extreme way I have so far, and she certainly doesn't like it. Her face flushes and starts to twist, as she considers what next to screech at me.

"Just stop and leave me alone, you complete maniac!" I yell into her sweaty, swollen face.

"Tramp. Fuck off and leave me alone, Tramp!" she rants, but I notice that she looks around to see if there are any witnesses. A van from the local council is parked on the opposite side of the road and the workmen are all leaning towards the open windows, queueing up for the best view of these two women arguing in the street.

"Leave me alone!" I yell again, turning to pick up the bag I dropped. Phoebe is standing hesitantly a few yards ahead, and I realise that it's far too dangerous to entertain Crazy Carolanne by the side of a busy road. My main concern right now is my dog's safety.

Carolanne steps away from me with her eyes on the council van. She looks scared, and this makes me feel good. "Can you see this?! Look at her!" I yell at the men and, as one, they all look at Carolanne. They had been looking at me in my tightfitting running gear and to be honest, I don't blame them. "She's been harassing and stalking me for weeks! Look at her face! I'm calling the fucking police!" As I shouted again, they had turned back to look at me. As if ordered, they turned back to Carolanne in unison, and it's almost funny. She spins on her heels and runs to where her car is parked. The men turn back to look at me and I point at her car. "Look at her! Look at her car! Police will call you as you are witnesses!" I'm closer to the van now and can lower my voice to seem more reasonable. "Ok?!"

One of the men nods, and the other two look shocked at a scene that has woken them up more than the contents of the Starbucks coffee cups littering the dashboard.

"Sure. No problem", says the one who nodded, so I smile my thanks and turn away, determined to take my dog for the run she was promised only a few minutes ago.

Walking briskly along the pier to the steps, I hear the familiar sound of Carolanne's car speeding up the hill out of the village. Even the bloody car sounds angry!

With witnesses now, she couldn't continue the assault as she would have liked. I think I hear a faint cry of "Fat cow" from her open window.

Once safely out of sight, I sit on the bottom step of the pier, dig my feet into the sand, and start to cry. Shaking in fear and confusion about why this woman is so determined to harm me in whatever way possible, I call the police.

This time, they can do something. Screaming and yelling abuse from her car or doorway is one thing. Heck, I deserve that, even if she doesn't know I do! But hitting me twice and putting my dog in danger in such a crazed way, all these weeks after we fell out, is frightening and... *out of control*. Her unpredictability, and disrespect for the law, is the most frightening thing about all this; I don't know what she might do next.

"Hey! Are you ok?!" Lauren's behind me.

"God sakes... of all the people to see now", I hiss at my feet and pretend to retie my shoelaces. Wiping my face on my sleeves, one by one, I hope I look vaguely collected.

"Was that Carolanne I saw driving away?" Lauren's stopped by my side, but I still can't look up to her face.

"Yes. It's been going on for weeks".

"Well, you were warned," Lauren's unsympathetic, but at least she doesn't sound as disgusted as she did the last time we were together. Remembering my friend's pale, shocked face, and how she ran from the meeting, makes me want to cry again. "Look, Lauren, we need to talk..."

"I don't want to talk about it just now. Not here anyway. She's probably still driving around looking for you. By the way, I haven't told anyone. I'm not going to tell anyone". Well! I'm not the only one who practised a speech for this meeting. Lauren goes on. "I just want a quiet life, and to try and get Oliver and I back on track. He's finally settled down. Says he wants kids!" Her voice is warmer now she's on her favourite subject.

She sits down next to me and I start talking. "At least with Jamie, I could predict what next and prepare for it. Carolanne is different. I think she's way past angry. I think she's actually a *sociopath*". Saying the last sentence out loud makes my chest thud.

"Well, she has form for being crazy, but you're the expert in these types. Especially after what happened to you before you came here". Lauren's voice has changed again, she sounds nice; like she used to.

"Do you want to go for a drive, maybe go for a drink?" I look up at her and the familiar scarf she wears brushes my cheek, and I recognise the flowery perfume she always wears. Closing my eyes to stop the tears again, I hold my breath. I'm waiting for Lauren to say no.

"Sure. He's not home for another few hours and, let's be honest, neither of us has a massive group of friends to pick and choose from!" Her familiar giggle makes me smile and the sun comes out - just a little.

"Go on, then. Tell me what happened. No details, just how the bloody hell you ended up doing THAT!" Lauren's flushed from too many white wines in the far-too-small pub we found about 30 miles along the coast. The drive was quiet, but it felt nice being with my friend again. Phoebe lay snoring on the back seat, glad of the relaxed atmosphere after that morning's roadside drama.

"Something's wrong with me. Well, definitely was wrong with me, back then. I've racked my brains trying to work out why or how it happened. It was just once, by the way. Just once. Straight away I felt bad. I hate myself", sipping the coke she bought me along with her own second glass of wine, I look away; embarrassed again.

"Well, you're clearly mortified. I would be!" She puts her hand on my shoulder and tries to tug me around to face her. "The Forgivers Club is for things like this. It's for people to share their darkest secrets and feel better. Lighter. More calm. Let's face it. People have done worse. Much worse than you, Lola".

She's being so nice and I'm so relieved I could burst with love for her. "Thank you for being so good about this. I've really missed you these last few weeks. Badly". She flushes with pleasure; she really is someone who needs someone. A wingman, a pal or buddy. She's like me. A lot.

We talk some more about what happened, and I blurt some things that I probably shouldn't have. Lauren's acceptance of my crime has me drunk on relief. As usual, my mouth races on and my brain doesn't catch up. I make her laugh a few times with my quips about being a Virgin-slayer and my expertise in the bedroom and, before I can stop myself, I've gone too far. The guilt washes over me again and I curse my big fat mouth and stupid need to impress people with humour, when it's absolutely not the time for it. I'm just so fucking glad we are friends again, and that she has accepted my mistake for just that - *a mistake*.

"Come on. Let's get you home. Oliver will be back soon, and I bet he's the type who likes his dinner on the table and his slippers by the fire!"

"Pfffft! Dinner yes, slippers no!" She chuckles and starts pulling her cardigan on, clumsily. Waving the sleeves to open them up, she staggers a little as we head towards the door.

"Yeah, well, he's lucky to have you. Let's go. I need to drop some clothes off at that seamstress I like. The one in that wee half village near Bridgefell? Up on the hill? I had to get some winter clothes. Never thought I'd stay nearly a whole year, and they need taking up *and* in!"

****

It's a few days later, and the wind has whipped itself into a bit of a frenzy; it's whirling around the bay, fast and hard. The sea's choppy and I think I can smell rain. The beach is empty and, in the late afternoon, it's starting to get a little gloomy down here on the shore.

"Let's go and collect those clothes, Pheebs!" I shout and she stops running away and turns to look at me. "I swear you understand me!" I say quietly, buttoning up my thin summer jacket to the top and tucking my scarf in a little tighter. I've forgotten my hat, and my hair - longer than it was when I arrived - catches in my eyes. "It's freezing. Let's go!" I shout and she starts to run back to me.

Laughing and running side by side until she easily overtakes me, we head towards my car parked on the jetty.

"Heater on. Music on. Let's go!" I cry, digging in my pockets for the car keys. The setting sun catches something on the side of the car. Expecting an errant bird poo or maybe a blade of grass, I reach out to wipe it away. My heart stops as I see what it really is; "Nice door Cow", it reads.

It's Carolanne. She's been here. Turning fast, almost slipping on the stone steps up of the jetty, my breath catches as I see her standing a few hundred yards away, leaning against her own car and smoking a roll-up cigarette. She waves at me slowly and grins her usual nasty grin.

It was only last week that I finally re-painted the door into my little flat. Previously it was a pale dusky blue, a favourite colour of Jen's. Now, with her permission, I've painted it a deep navy blue, like the sea early in the morning. It's a message; Carolanne's reminding me she's not just watching me, but that she's responsible for the damage to both the door to my home and, now, my car.

Running my fingers along the scratched words, 2-foot-high, into the car's bonnet, I feel anger start to ripple through me. She's going too far now. No matter what, I don't deserve this. It's been nearly four months! She has no idea about Sam and me, and she's acting completely evil. Deliberate, sustained, planned, stalking and harassment.

"Fucking nutter!" I yell as she spins in the car park and drives away up the hill. The music she has always plays too loud, fades off as she turns the corner and disappears from sight.

****

"I'm afraid there's not enough evidence for us to do anything, really". The officer is trying to look like he cares. It's the same one I reported the damage to my door to; again. He arrived the day after Carolanne scratched my car and I reported the incident, his excuse being "very busy" in this traditionally crimefree part of the country.

"Is there anyone else I can speak to? That's ridiculous. She's chased me, attacked me, constantly called and messaged, and now these two sets of vandalism which are clearly linked!"

"It's irrelevant. They will say the same as me. We need evidence. Same as last time. Two pieces and, sadly, your dog can't talk", he laughs at his own stupid, pointless, joke. "Just forget it then! She's escalating! Getting worse! And, when she kill's me, will you be bothered then?!"

"If there are two pieces of evidence that she did it, then yes, we will, Miss Hague. Of course", he picks his hat up off the table and stands slowly, readying himself to leave. He's only been here nine minutes. I know, because I've counted.

Each time the police come now, I make a note of how long they stay, note down their excuses for doing nothing, and keep a log of the incident number they eagerly give me, with that being the sum of all the work they are prepared to do. Labelling each incident, separately, going against actual proper Stalking and Harassment law enforcement guidelines. I know, because these last few weeks I've made myself an expert in it. Jen's computer in the deli's office has been almost as close a friend as Lauren.

"Fine. See you soon, I'm sure of it. She's not going to stop. It's what she does. People around here have told me". Trevenna reddens a little, but turns away fast.

"Like I said, we welcome all reports of possible crime and will do all we can, whenever we can, Miss Hague. Have a nice evening".

I slam the door at his back and watch as he walks easily to the police car. He's been to see me about Carolanne 11 times now. "Idiot", I mutter, wrapping my apron right around my increasingly-slim frame. "That reminds me. We need to go and pick those clothes up, Pheebs. In fact, I could do with some fresh air. Let's go now".

"Your friend picked the clothes up the other day". The seamstress is smiling benignly at me like the words actually make sense.

"What?! No. My friend hasn't picked them up! She's in the car, waiting for me". I'd offered Lauren a trip out, unsure about being on my own, and afraid of being targeted by Carolanne again.

"Well, a different friend then". The seamstress looks a bit cross, or maybe embarrassed, now. "Either way, she said she was your friend; she described you, and they're gone. She took them. For you". She points at me and waggles her finger left then right as she says the last two words. I'm speechless but understanding floods upwards from my feet to my mouth, fast.

"What did she look like. This woman. Tell me!"

The seamstress steps away from the desk, looking panicked at my manic reaction to this seemingly silly situation. "Calm down! Well, she wasn't like you, that's for sure. She was taller, long brown, dark brown hair, and older. A bit older, yes"

Pleased as punch at her detailed description, the seamstress steps away from the counter and sits back down at the sewing machine furthest from the counter. "Was she local? Local accent?"

"Sure! In fact, I think I know her face. That's why I was fine giving her them. Locals wouldn't go around nicking clothes for no reason. Too small around here. Too easy to get caught". The sewing machine whirrs into life. The conversation is over.

****

Lauren's driving and I'm on the phone shouting and crying at the police officer on the other end. "You have to do something now! That's a witness! Maybe CCTV too. In the street. Her car outside. Her face. Accent. All of it. That's it. You can arrest her. Stop her. Help me now!" He's quiet at the other end and it unnerves me. "Hello! Hello!"

"I'm still here, Miss Hague. Let me see what I can do. I'll get back to you in due course". Then the phone goes dead. "This is what she wants, Lola. You all messed up and upset. In a state. It's why she does it". Lauren's slowed the car down so she can hand me a tissue. The roads are winding and, even at this time of year, tourists are common with their city-driving ways, and need for speed to see a sunset or sunrise before anyone else.

"I think she's sending me crazy! I can't handle all this. I just left someone who made me bonkers, and now this mad creature?! It makes no sense unless she really is just fixated on me. Gay or jealous or bored or all of these things! Bloody hell, the clothes are three, no four sizes too small for her!" Wailing into the tissue all the way home does me no good, and I spend the rest of the night awake, researching ways to stop this woman ruining my life - no, my sanity, all over again.

* * * * * * * * * * * * *

It's a few days later and I have been eagerly waiting to see what comes of the clothing theft. I feel hope that this is it; the chance I have to finally get some sort of real police intervention.

Trevenna looks bored before he even speaks. "Tell me some good news. Please". I sit down opposite him and lean forward expectantly. Then he hits me with yet more disappointment.

"Nothing we can do about it. I went to see the woman in the shop, and she says she can't positively identify who took your clothes. Couldn't give a name. Good news, though! I have them here for you, if you want them!" I stare at the officer as he thrusts a carrier bag at me. It's a plastic bag from the local shop here in Bridgefell. I'd put my clothes into the seamstress in a paper bag. A pretty patterned one, from Padstow.

"Now the clothes are back, it's not even really a crime. Just a silly mistake!" He smiles but his eyes slide away towards the door. My mouth falls open in dismay as Trevenna slaps his knees and stands up. This time he hasn't even been here long enough to take his hat off.

"That's it?" My voice is weak and husky from the previous night's lack of sleep and too much wine.

"Looks like it. Keep your head down and things will settle themselves down. I'm sure of that!" Trevenna's gone as fast as usual, and I sit in the bistro office chair for the next hour, crying.

"None of this makes sense!" I sob, as Lauren waits patiently at the end of the phone a few hours later.

"I admit, she is a bit extra crazy over you. I've seen her bad and heard rumours, but she's deffo obsessed with you, that's for sure!"

"I just want her to leave me alone. I'm ill with it all. I can't go on like this. Do you know, at the beginning, way back in August, one of her messages read that she hoped I would die? That I should kill myself!"

Lauren gasps but says nothing. "I know! Right?! That was the very first night she started. *I hope you kill yourself*. That's what she said. She might just get her bloody wish at this rate!"

Listen to: *Wilson Phillips – Hold On*

Chapter 14: Warnings

It's been easy to self-isolate. A lot easier than I expected. Carolanne's poisoned darts have struck quite a few necks in the village, and there are fewer and fewer invitations "around for tea" or "out for a drink" as each week slides by. Jamie taught me how to be wary of other people, and yet I still made the mistake of befriending the local sociopath! "Well done, Lola", I mutter, and the words are torn up by the wind.

It's early November and the sea-air is bitterly cold, especially on these days without a cloud in the sky. Phoebe's racing ahead and fighting the breeze; her tongue lolling and little fat legs struggling, she's loving every minute of this early winter morning.

"Lola!" Kay's voice soars past on the wind and for a second, I think it's just gulls calling to each other but she shouts to me again, making me stop walking even though I don't want to see her, or anybody, today.

Especially low and fearful, I know I look drawn and pale. In fact, looking at me you'd know I'm weighed down with regret and shame. I'm so filled up with it that I can't eat, and so pressed down to the bed with it that I can't sleep.

"Hey! How've you been!?" She's jogging towards me and looks unusually upbeat.

"Not great" I reply, and turn away to make sure Phoebe's still in sight. She's wrestling with a stick of seaweed a few yards away; her tail straight up and ears straight back in determination to "kill" it, fast and furiously. She'll need a bath when we get home.

"Can I walk with you a bit?" Kay's taken my arm without waiting for my reply.

Walking to the steps onto the street twenty minutes later, I'm glad Kay found me after all. "If you need anyone to talk to you, know where I am, ok?" she hugs me and backs away. "Call me later!" she shouts ,and turns to skip up the steps. Watching her go, I realise how important it is that I do talk to someone about what happened; about what I did. Fit to burst, I'm ready to call the police myself, but Kay had talked me out of it only a few minutes ago.

"Look at the way she is now, and she has no idea about Sam and you! You can't tell her, or anyone else, Lola! She'll kill you both!"

"I know, but I feel like I'm dead already and this is no life. She's making it Hell for no reason as it is, and I'm worried about Phoebe; to be honest, her lack of consistency and constant changing ways to get at me have made me as ill as I was when I came here... *worse even*".

"Well. You know my opinion, and I'm older and wiser than you!" she'd said, and squeezed me close, as a strengthening wind caught our faces. "Let's walk back".

Sitting on the wall surrounding the beach and thinking about Kay's words, I'm startled by the familiar tooting of Carolanne's car horn. "Oi! You!" She's yelling from the car and waving at Kay. Shrinking back against the wall, sliding down out of sight, I can see what happens next although I can't hear it.

Kay and Carolanne exchange words; starting angry then easing into friendly. I watch them share the last of Carolanne's cigarette and talk for a few minutes. Kay had told me she had no intention of breaking what minor friendship she already had with Carolanne, for fear of "repercussions" similar to the ones I was experiencing.

"Best to let her think she's the boss and she's in control. Might be wimpy, but it works. Years of watching her in action makes me an expert in how to handle her bags-full of crazy", she'd texted me a few days after my confession at The Forgivers Club.

This looks and feels different though; like they are comfortable with each other. Kay turns abruptly as if she can feel me watching, and I shrink further onto the sand, holding Phoebe tightly to me. Breathing heavily, I know something just passed between the two women, and it's something not good for me or my safety here. Kay looked angry and not with Carolanne.

****

"Hi, Lola. Erm, it's best you don't come in here anymore", the barmaid whispers harshly. Gently pulling me by my sleeve towards the end of the bar, and looking to see who's watching, she hands my ten-pound note back and closes my hand into a fist around it.

It's a few days since I saw Kay on the beach, and I've taken myself out for a drink to a small pub I've discovered since the incident with Steph.

"What do you mean, not come here anymore? Why?" My heart's beating out of rhythm, but I know the answer before she gives it to me. "We've had some nasty calls, and even a bad review on the pub website. A person saying you're a prostitute and a man-stealer… that was the exact phrasing. I can't take the risk of any trouble, and the person's been in touch with the brewery too…"

She's red in the face and I can see sweat pools in the baggy grey t-shirt she's worn every time I've been here. "I can guess who it is, who's making trouble for you… It's ok". Putting the ten-pound note in the charity box on the bar, and almost enjoying watching the barmaid cringe in shame, my last words are louder than she wanted. "Funny how people are loyal to faceless trolls and not actual paying customers, isn't it?!"

****

I'm still red with humiliation 30 minutes later. Walking home along the clifftop, I start to feel dangerously angry. Carolanne's had her time making me miserable! During and after our fall-out, for devils' sakes! I've a choice to make. Confess what happened with Sam, take my punishment properly from a court, she's still going to be evil; or keep the secret, struggle with it, and remain a target of hers anyway.

"Thing is, she's losing her own victimhood-status the more she carries on! People have to see how deranged she is, whether I'm the monster or not!" I yell at the sea, and the waves below seem to crash in reply; angrier than me, if that's even possible.

The only thing stopping me handing myself in and confessing, is worry about what will happen to Phoebe. She's my baby, my child, my whole world, sad as that may be.

"Just you wait there; I'll be back in two minutes, Pheebs". Tying her lead around the same lamppost I always do, I check the street for any sign of Carolanne before heading inside the garage shop. It's dark outside, and I've just popped out for some milk and eggs; I'm trialling a new cherry and chocolate tart for the deli, and excited that Jen and Louise are back in a few days' time, just for a swift check-up on things.

My neck prickles and, without even thinking, I back away from the counter to look through the window to check on Phoebe. I can usually see her tail from this position although, right now, there's nothing. My chest thuds and I drop the eggs and milk. Swinging the door open I'm faced with Carolanne, on her knees, untying my dog and smiling nastily. She looks up and the smile slides off her face, illuminated by the lights from the shop and the wet pavement at her feet. She looks evil; she *is* evil.

"Get the fuck away from my dog!" I yell, and start to shake with the adrenalin-shot of fear. She stands up slowly. "You're paranoid, Homewrecker. Maybe you should watch your dog, and your back, more carefully".

Phoebe snakes between my feet and I can feel her shaking. "Carolanne. This has to stop. YOU have to stop. It's been months. This isn't normal!" I'm trying to reason with her, and my own soft voice makes me want to cry. Why can't she just leave me alone and get on with her life?

"Nah. You deserve it", she says, tossing her hair and walking down the street towards the pub, her hands in the pockets of the army camo jacket she always wears. "Bye, bitch!" she yells, and disappears from sight, around the corner.

"What was that all about?!" The shopkeeper's behind me. "Bring the dog inside. It's against shop rules, but you look like you need a few minutes". Sitting down in the back office of the shop, I break down and tell the shopkeeper, Brian, everything that's happened since I came to the village, and even some things about why I came here in the first place.

"Well, I'm a witness now, so when you call the police, you can give them my details and surely then she'll stop. I've had a few run-ins with her myself. Nothing huge, but she likes to throw her weight about, that one. The milk's off when it's not, so she gets it free of charge. The cigarettes were missing three fags, so I gave them her free of charge. Once she even sent her son in here, 70p short of a pack of bacon. Felt sorry for the lad, I did".

At his reference to Sam, I buckle over and wail all over again. This man wouldn't be so nice if he knew what I did. "Well, I'll call the police tomorrow, Brian. They've been useless so far. If I didn't know better, I'd say she has some hold over them, or there's a reason they won't charge her or deal with her properly".

Brian steps away from me quickly and busies himself tidying an impeccable row of tins. "If I were you, I wouldn't mention anything like that again. To anyone, missy. Take my advice. Loose talk like that won't do you any favours around here. Small places have big secrets", he whispers the last sentence between cupped hands, not breaking eye contact. It's almost theatrical and makes me laugh.

"Oh, you have no idea, Brian. No idea at all!"

"Get yourself off home. Here's a bottle of wine on the house, as they say. You'll need it. Tired as an old rag, you look, and that dog is a nervous wreck. Daft, the pair of you!"

Walking out to the chime of the shop bell, I turn and wave at Brian who's standing at the window watching me go safely. "Mind what I said!" he calls, and I wave back although, admittedly, I do feel uneasy. Practically running the few hundred yards up the street and to home, I keep looking over my shoulder for Carolanne and her familiar car.

* * * * * * * * * * * * * * *

"Right. We've spoken to Brian from the shop and indeed, he is happy to sign a statement to the effect of a breach of the peace last night". Officer Trevenna doesn't look exactly keen or happy that we have finally got Carolanne banged to rights. "However…" he coughs, and my heart sinks. "It's going to be a breach of the peace, and not attempted theft as I know you are hoping for". Now he smiles a little and it unnerves me.

"Why?! It's on the CCTV, and with all the other stuff, and what she actually said about me watching myself and my dog more carefully. Surely you can get a harassment charge or something more serious!" He squirms in his seat and tucks the notepad away.

"Unfortunately not, Miss Hague. Take what you can get in this instance. She was very silly to make such a statement in public in the first place".

"Silly?! Silly?! Are you mental?!" Standing up I lean back against the deli counter and fold my arms, desperate to hold in the shouts of rage and accusations of police misconduct I know won't help right now.

"Miss Hague. Please calm down. This is a small community, and we can't go arresting everyone you allege are upsetting you. I've told you she will be charged and referred to the CPS for Breach of the Peace. Now take that, and run with it as you like. Either way, I have things to be getting on with. Going to see Carolanne, for a start off".

"There's something not right about all this", I yell as he walks out onto the street. His back stiffens and he stops. Turning around slowly, he pins me with steely blue eyes and leans back into the shop, right into my own personal space. His breath is warm on my face.

"Be careful what you accuse people of around here, Lola" he whispers, and I recoil. Now I know for sure there's something going on underneath all this. He's given the game away by trying to protect her, or whatever it is she knows, now.

"Do I look like the sort of person to stay quiet, Officer?!" Not breaking eye contact, I can feel the mistake spreading through me, but I can't stop. "I'm going to make a formal complaint about how you are dealing with her, and I'm not going to leave it until she leaves me alone and you do what you're paid to do. I might not be a local exactly, but there's a limit to the hell anyone can put another person through day... after... DAY!" I yell the last word as he was walking away to the front of the police car the whole time I was speaking.

"Like I said, I'm going to see her now. The CPS will be in touch with whatever decision they take as, once she leaves my station later, she's all theirs".

He deftly reverses the car and turns, driving clumsily up onto the pavement as he goes. "That's a driving an offence, you know!" I yell as he disappears out of sight.

Half an hour later I've made a decision. There's no way I'm going to report myself for what happened with Sam. It's gone way past me being the bad guy now. She's messed with me too much and for too long, and my own guilt now barely reaches the sides in comparison to how furious I am at her constant abuse these last few months; as far as she is aware, it's actually all been for nothing.

"She doesn't deserve my confession. Not anymore!" I rant, kneading bread dough vigorously. "It's gone too far now. Far,

far too far and I have a feeling that, whatever happens, I'm going to be treated badly and unfairly. There's something going on here with her and that cop. Maybe more people involved. This place is starting to stink!"

That's the problem with thinking you're above the law, and you can make someone's life a misery, just for fun. One day, the target of your hate starts to get angry and then you have two wrongs making absolutely nothing right...

Listen to: *Cher – If I Could Turn Back Time*

Chapter 15: Burnt

"Any excuse for a bonfire around here!" Lauren crows and tugs me towards the huge flaming pyre.

"Well, it is Guy Fawkes, Lauren!" Laughing, I tug my arm back. "Let's get some food and have a quick scan about. Make sure Carolanne isn't here. She'd happily push me in that fire as quick as you can say firework!"

Lauren and I weave through the throbbing crowd mostly made up of tourists. A few familiar faces here and there smile and nod at us, sip at drinks, and then carry on their conversations. No one invites us to join them. "Looks like she's done the rounds pretty successfully. I'm now the local pariah and yet not a reason for it... yet!" I say loudly enough for just Lauren to hear over the crackling fire and chatter of people around us.

"Ssshhhhhhh, Lola. Don't get too cocky. Folk might seem disinterested in you but they're always watching, even when you think they aren't". Lauren hands me a drink.

"Fair enough. Funny though. That Brian chap from the garage shop said something similar actually". I'm a bit tipsy from the bottle of wine that we'd already shared in the flat, and the heat of the fire's making me woozy.

"Oh look! There's Oliver!" Lauren squeals. My chest hurts but I've no intention of making a scene by going home just because he's here. It's been weeks since the beach party and Lauren deserves a little social-loyalty, after all this time supporting me.

"Ok, but I can't stay long. Phoebe's good with fireworks when I'm there but on her own in the flat, she'll be going nuts.

Jen's back tomorrow and last thing I need is a wet carpet or scratches on the wall to explain away!"

As Lauren pulls me across the field towards the familiar shape of Oliver with, I think, Rob next to him, I catch sight of Sam on the other side of the fire. He raises his plastic cup and nods at me but doesn't smile. Behind him, his mother appears and sees him looking at me. She grabs him and pulls him backwards into a group of people and he disappears from view.

"Hey, babe!" Lauren jumps on Oliver's back and he swings her around doing a fantastic job of being glad to see her. He winks at me and I look away, finishing my drink. Rob starts to walk towards me, mouth open, full of some bullshit as usual.

"I'm going to get another drink, see you in 10". I yell in Lauren's direction as she's being swung left and right, and is screeching in glee. Oliver's extremely drunk, and I wish I hadn't let her drag me over here.

"Don't, Robert. I've no time or patience for you right now", he stops walking at my raised hands and his face falls. I feel almost guilty, but not enough to stay around for his crap about Horseface, and what she's done now to trigger yet another breakup binge.

Wandering towards the bar tent, I can't help but look out for Kay; we haven't spoken since our short walk on the beach last week, and something's niggling me about how she interacted with Carolanne. She seemed comfortable; more so than I expected considering how "afraid of her wrath" as she twice described herself.

I'm cautious about giving into the paranoia, but with Carolanne's' persistent stalking and almost daily disturbances, I can't help but wonder how far she'd go to not only run me out of the village, but ruin whatever I build, wherever I go. The way she's pushed around anyone who's supported me, and even isolated me from the pub in the other village, tells me this woman has no boundaries and plenty of ideas up her sleeve left to come.

People certainly aren't as friendly as they were when I first arrived and there is a distinct cooling of the atmosphere even now, beside the huge roaring bonfire. Standing alone, sipping the mulled wine I donated to the event, with no one bothering to come over and say Hi, it's pretty clear Carolanne's' poison is spreading.

There's a presence to my left and, cup raised to my lips, I turn slowly to see Oliver's defiant jaw as he stands a little too close and watches the flames. "Look, Oliver, I don't want any trouble". Stepping away to create a foot of space between us, I button my coat up higher.

"Neither do I. Seems like you're no longer in a position to pick and choose your mates though, Lola. Not now. Not after what you did". He turns to look at me and smiles nastily. My chest freezes and the mulled wine rises up, threatening to make a reappearance.

"And what do you mean by that, exactly?" I already know but I want to hear him say it.

"Sam". That name, that one word and the ground at my feet tilts. Oliver reaches out to steady me but holds my arm a little too tightly. "Lauren has a big mouth when she's got a drink in her. Shame you don't know her as well as you think. You've not been here long enough to see beneath her pretty face and puppy-dog eyes. When she wants something, she will sell out anyone and anything to get it".

"And she wants *you*", I whisper, not taking my eyes off his.

"Yep. She's desperate to put me... off you, so sharing your filthy secret was her way of doing it. Well, she thinks it's worked. But. of course, it hasn't. You are every teenage boy's dream and every man's fantasy, Lola". Oliver leans forward and winks at me, still holding my arm.

"Oliver, whatever you think you're doing right now, don't do it". Tugging my arm away, I take a step backwards but bump into someone who swears and grunts "Idiot" at me. I need to go home. Gather my thoughts. Work out how to deal with this new threat.

"I think you need to go home. I'll walk you". He takes my arm and throws the rest of my drink into the fire. He starts to guide me gently but firmly through the crowd towards the gate, and the road back to the village.

"I can get myself home, thank you, Oliver. Lauren will see you're missing and come looking for you, anyway". I tug my arm uselessly as he tightens his grip and walks faster.

"She's plastered anyway. 10 minutes won't hurt", he hisses under his breath.

It's quiet now we're away from the fire; darker too. "Oliver, I'll scream if you touch me!" I make an attempt at firm, but my voice is shaky. This is all far, far, too familiar. Stumbling on the wet and boggy grass, I have to hold onto him to stop myself falling. Once on the ground, he'll have more opportunity so I can't let myself trip up. The mulled wine was strong; I added brandy to it and, on an empty stomach, it's quickly making an impact.

"You won't make a fuss, Lola. The last thing you need is attention and people asking questions, isn't it?" he whispers this in my ear, even though there's now not a soul in sight.

"Likewise. Your girlfriend will murder the pair of us if we're seen together, and you won't get a chance to explain you were blackmailing me to get me here". Pulling and tugging. I can't get free then he suddenly lets go and I fall backwards into the mud.

He looms over me blocking out the light of the moon, and I hear the zipper of his flies as he opens them. Flashes of Jamie and what he used to do, just suddenly demanding sex or something else rush past, and a surge of hate takes me by surprise, quick enough for me reach my right harm back, make a fist and punch out, straight into Oliver's crotch. He makes a squealing sound like air released from a balloon and falls back himself into the mud, against the gate.

"Men like you should be castrated at birth, and I've seen more than my fair share, mate", I whisper in his ear as he curls into a foetal position and moans what sounds like "fucking paedo bitch".

"Funny you're calling me that now when you were just about to rape me. Let's keep this a secret, shall we? I know a club you can join if the burden gets too much". I'm clambering over him, and then quickly swing my legs over the gate. Once on the other side and trying to neaten myself up, just in case a car drives past or someone has seen us, I realise how muddy and stained with grass I am.

He'd pushed me into a very dangerous situation; a situation I very nearly didn't get out of. "Fucking hell. There's something wrong with you, Oliver. Really, really wrong. I was raped when I was 17, by two older men. Do you know that? Lauren didn't share that, did she? No. I bet not. She doesn't want you to feel sorry for me, never mind fancy me!"

"Lola", he mutters and moans again.

"Nah. Fuck you!" I shout, already running towards the village. It starts to rain and, fleetingly, I hope he drowns in the mud; like the pig he is.

Less than 10 minutes later, I'm rounding the corner at the top of the village. It's deserted, everyone else is at the bonfire. Stopping to take a few deep breaths, I sit on the bench overlooking the streets below. Only yesterday I sat here with Phoebe, sketching the view. I'd had an idea to sketch different scenes of the village to individualise the menus in the bistro, as a surprise for Jen and Louise. A sob escapes. I'm trapped here. I can't let Jen down and just leave. And I have to face it, wherever I go, Carolanne's going to haunt me.

A light goes on in the bistro and my heart thuds; they're back early. No, my watch says half 10. "Fuck". How the hell am I going to explain the mess I'm in? "Drunk enough to fall in mud" is embarrassing, and Jen's not going to leave me in charge of her business if I'm the type to do that. "Oliver Moon tried to rape me as a sort of blackmail plot, because he found out I had sex with Sam, a week before his 16th birthday" sounds a tad worse. "Let's go with the drunk story, Lola",

I mutter, walking quickly down the hill. "At least that's believable".

Walking into the bistro car park, I can see more lights flicking on, and then Jen's voice as she finds Phoebe. It makes me want to cry again; her lovely, familiar, motherly, voice and how glad she is to be home and seeing us. "Get it together, Lola. You can do this".

"Hi! Welcome home!" I cry opening the front door and walking straight into the café; a smile plastered on, and a prayer under my breath that I don't look as bad as I think I do.

"What the hell happened to you?!" Jen embraces me and I catch sight of Louise behind her. She slowly folds her arms and leans back against the counter. "Hello, both! You look super-tanned! Lucky sods! Let me get cleaned up and make you something to eat. The bonfire got a bit rowdy, and folk were pushing and shoving a bit to see the fireworks. Of course, I was the first in the mud, but judging by the zombie apocalypse crowd behind me, heading home, I wasn't the last!" Refusing eye contact, I slip past Louise and leave Jen staring speechless after me.

Showering the mud off and blocking the plughole with dirt and grass, I turn the water up to its highest setting to muffle my cries. But I don't think it covers up Phoebe's whining at the bathroom door.

Listen to: Radio Head – Creep

Chapter 16: She Said, She Said

"Are you free for a chat? Maybe a walk, too?" The message is read but not replied to by Lauren. She's most likely hungover, and stuck to Oliver; desperate not to, as usual, let him out of her sight. I don't even know why I want to see her. I've no intention of telling her what happened the other day, but I do want to ask her who else she's told my secret to.

Anxiety is rippling through me, making my hands shake constantly. Jen noticed it today when I was trying to ice some fairy cakes. "You're a wreck, Lola! It's like you were when you came here!" She's holding both of my hands palm up, and frowning at them.

"Too much coffee as usual, Jen. Don't worry about me". I pull my hands free and turn away, and start cutting tiny leaves from the green icing I rolled out earlier.

"You do seem rattled, Lola". Louise's deeper voice comes from the doorway. She's not worried though; her face is flat and expressionless. "If there's something you need to tell us, now's a good time". She sits herself at the table nearest the counter where her wife and I are working. She crosses her legs and finishes the last of the espresso I left there earlier. Stress is making me forgetful, too.

"Nope, nothing at all, ladies. Honestly! Now you're back for a bit, can we try out some more of my ideas for the winter menu? And, as usual, this place is doing the starters and desserts for the Village Christmas Fayre which is…" Busying myself with the calendar hanging above the till, I can feel Louise's stare on my neck. She never liked me; that much was clear from the start. "… next week. The Sunday".

The bell signalling the bistro door opening and shutting makes me jump. "Ignore her. She's fed up already, and wants us back in Portugal as soon as", Jen says, rubbing my back. "Show me your ideas, and I love the menu designs". Jen kisses my cheek and guides me to the table we use for our "meetings".

****

Padstow's busier than I expected; laden down with shopping bags, I'm trying to navigate the narrow streets and get back to the car before the rain starts. Head down slightly, I'm not watching where I'm going. I should've worn a hat; it's absolutely freezing now with December around the corner.

There are fairy lights strung up above the streets nearest the town centre, giving the town a magical aura. "No wonder it's busy. Must be the nicest way to shop in the whole of Cornwall", a man's voice whispers from behind. Spinning a bit too fast, I catch him on the knees with my shopping bags, and he winces as he steps back. "Or maybe not!" he laughs, rubbing his legs and winking at me, before putting his hands in his coat pockets. He's attractive; older than me. A lot older, actually, but that doesn't detract from how good-looking he is. Not at all.

"Yeah, well. You can't go around creeping up on people". My embarrassment has me bad-tempered, a default reaction that needs a lot more work. "Sorry. I don't mean to be so nippy. I got a wee fright there". Blushing and hot as Hell now, I take a deep breath and prepare to apologise properly. "I don't do surprises and I'm a bit tense. Crowds and noise make me edgy. It's not your fault, it's mine".

He's smiling and not talking, and it's unnerving me. In fact, I think he's enjoying my embarrassment. He has nice eyes, a sort of grey-green, I think. Lots of hair for someone maybe in their late 40s or early 50's, and he's dressed nicely. Unusual for around here, where its farmer chic or surfer dude, and not much else in between. "You're massive", the words are out before I can stop them.

"Ok! Well it's been a while since anyone pointed it out quite so... bluntly. Yes, I'm 6ft 3, 4. You'd need to ask my mum or maybe measure me yourself", he laughs. "But I think you'd need a step ladder, as you're tiny!" My turn to laugh and I realise we're flirting. "Coffee?" he says taking the heaviest of the bags from my feet.

"Tea", I reply, handing him the other bag and smiling.

It's been an age since I flirted with anyone, especially sober and harmlessly. And this is harmless. I don't know him, and he doesn't have a ring on. Not to mention, he hasn't sent me a picture of his knob yet, or demanded one of my boobs. The thought makes me smile. Maybe there are decent men in the world; mind you, there's still time for him to ruin it, or me to mess up, for that matter.

The café windows are steamed up with the cold outside and over-populated tables inside, and Ben's watching me closely as I ram another coffee muffin in my mouth. "No wonder you're so small! You clearly don't eat. No appetite at all", he hands me a napkin and rocks back in his chair.

"Funny guy", I manage to say, although it's a risk considering how much cake I've still to swallow.

"While you're incapacitated, I'm going to ask you to simply nod at this next question". I know what's coming but I can't say yes; this incredibly nice, kind, and smart person can't be anywhere near my totally messed-up life.

"Are you shopping here again tomorrow?" He's clever, I'll give him that. I nod and swallow a bit more cake. "Are you single?" I nod again, but hope he doesn't ask me out; the thought makes me sad. Suddenly I feel sick, and tears threaten to ruin the goodbye I have to say as quickly as possible.

"Are you trouble? You look like trouble". At least this time I can nod and it's the truth. Sam's face, then Carolanne's voice, make me close my eyes against the shame I desperately want to share with Ben. Scare him off, and make this easy for me. For us both.

"Perfect" He says simply, and I watch as he takes my phone and puts his number in.

"It's not good trouble, though. Not good or fun or anything like that". I'm trying to say it without saying it. Gutless as ever.

"Can't be that bad!" He hands me my phone back and stands up. "I'd walk you back to your car but it's later than I thought. Your phone says half 5!" Shit. I was supposed to be home almost an hour ago. There's no time to explain or talk more, and relief tugs at my gut.

"Text or call me later, or tomorrow. Whatever suits". A quick kiss on the cheek and he's gone.

"Lucky Lady". The waitress has appeared as if by magic and is wiping the table. "You've done well there. Batten down the hatches for the influx of local women baying for your blood!" She giggles and walks away before I can reply "Yeah, well, nothing new there then!". Probably best, my cheeky and far too honest mouth only gets me in trouble these days, anyway.

****

"We need to talk". My phone lights up and for a split second I think it's him; he's already changed his mind. "Walk tomorrow?" No, it's Kay. I've not heard from her in days, almost a fortnight.

"I was beginning to think you were avoiding me", I send back; desperate for her to deny it and call me paranoid, I'm disappointed when she doesn't message back.

The beach is deserted which isn't a surprise, considering the snow coming down thick and fast. Phoebe's not as excited as usual and she walks slowly next to me, slightly hunched against the cold. She never has liked cold weather, and snow in particular is her least favourite. "Won't be long, Pheebs. Quick walk. Quick chat and home". She looks up at me and wanders off towards a mop-head of seaweed that looks (and smells) interesting.

A figure's walking towards me through the snow, and it takes me a few seconds to recognise Kay. She's not waving and, as she gets closer, I see she's not smiling either; my chest tightens in dread. "Hey! Who knew the weather would turn like this? I know it was cold, but snow?! It's mad, isn't it?" I call towards her, but she doesn't speak. This is bad.

"If I were you, I'd get packed up and leave, Lola. No one wants you here now". The words hit me straight in the face. Speechless and numb-faced from the cold, I don't know what to say. "I know what you did with Oliver. I saw you. At the bonfire". She's blunt, to the point, but so very, very wrong.

"It's not what you think. Let me explain". I reach for her, but she steps back. Glaring at me, she just keeps going.

"I saw you holding on to each other and head into the shadows, then disappear. He came back to the bonfire zipping himself up, and said you'd gone home. He was pleased as punch". Feeling faint I reach for her again, but she keeps moving. The beach is moving, too. Waves are crashing, but it's a calm day.

"No, no, no!" I can't seem to get the words out. Explain it right.

"They said - people said you were a homewrecker, but your best friend's man?! Really? When you really have no one else?! Even with what happened with my husband and that whore he left me for, I stood by you. I believed in you. I trusted you!"

She's shouting now and red-faced. Rooted to the spot I just stand there. "The Sam thing was bad but this, this is way worse!" She's in my space now; yelling and waving her arms around. Phoebe trots over to see what all the fuss is about, but settles at my feet instead of seeing Kay for some affection, like she usually does.

"Get packed and leave. Lauren's on the warpath and I'm beyond livid. It's dangerous for you here, now". She turns and walks quickly, along the beach, to where I can see her car parked next to mine.

I start running after her and shouting for her to stop, but whether she hears me or not, she doesn't stop. I'm faster than her, younger, fitter, but not fuelled by rage like she is; it takes me a good 10 seconds to catch her. "Kay! You've got it wrong!" I reach her and pull at the hem of her coat.

She turns and spits at me, full on in the face. Shocked and disgusted, I recoil and stumble back a little, standing on Phoebe's paw in the process. She yelps but Kay doesn't flinch.

"Carolanne's told me everything. About how you took your ex off some poor woman! You've come here saying he abused you, but you stole him from the woman you've said was involved! She and Carolanne have been talking for weeks. Carolanne tracked down the guy. She says he's lovely and so is the woman he's with! The one who says you stole him from her!"

"No, no, no! He told me he was single! Chased me for months! I didn't know she even existed until she started stalking me, and then he cheated on me with her, and then I found out..."

"Save it. I'm done with all your lies and dramas. It's disgusting. I knew it when you came here all blonde, and ditsy, and eager to please. I knew it! I ignored people saying what you really were, and even supported your miserable whining about Sam! I'm done and believe me when I say it, you are *done, too*!"

He's found me. She's found me, too. It's begun. The lies. The reputational damage. My truth doesn't matter. In the clamour of everyone else's bullshit, the truth just loses its power in the end. The hellfire I left behind has spread, and Carolanne's poison is fanning the flames. This is worse than I ever could have imagined.

Falling to my knees in the sand, I stay there until I find the strength to get up. Kay's car is long gone. Phoebe is next to me, shaking with fear and cold.

Listen to: Meat Loaf - Paradise By The Dashboard Light

Chapter 17: Trapped Again

The smart rat-a-tat of the rarely-used lion doorknocker for the shop downstairs makes me stop dead. "She's here", I whisper. A cold, quiet emptiness settles over me.

In a strange robotic state, I put Phoebe's collar on and lock her in the bathroom with a note to feed her five small meals a day, water and sometimes milk, and one walk a day is plenty. The knocking gets more persistent, but I don't move any faster; I don't want to panic Phoebe any more than she already is.

"Wait here. Mummy'll be back soon", I whisper into her fur and gently nudge her away from the door, shutting it without having the guts to look at her. Now, the tears start to clog my throat, but I know it's pointless. Crying and begging won't make a difference. I'm dead; it's that simple.

"Police. Lola!? It's the police. You need to let us in within a count of ten or we have the right to use a ram to force the door open, and no one wants that. Not at this time of the morning anyway". It's the same officer who was here the other day. Relief floods through me; rather him than her all day, any day of the week.

"Lola Hague, we're here to arrest you on suspicion of a sexual offence against a child…". I stop listening then. Deaf to whatever else the female officer says while the other one stands behind her, time slows down. I'm going to jail for a very long time, and I deserve it.

****

"Take your clothes off and put them there", a female police officer with thick brown hair is speaking gently and pointing to a chair at her side.

"Why?!" I'm shaking and even that one simple word takes three syllables.

"We have to take photographs of any distinguishing marks in case you decide to disappear once we let you go". She looks at me flatly, like I'm stupid. Like I should know this is the process for registering sex offenders. I'm a sex offender.

I want to slap myself in the face and wake up from this nightmare; go backwards sliding back up that hill, back up the motorway, away from this village. Away back home to the safer, easier Hell than this is going to be, once I set foot outside the station.

"You're letting me go?" I stop unbuttoning my denims and stare at her then the other, slimmer, dark blonde officer. She's more lined and has a meaner face, like she's done this a thousand times before, and hates every minute of it. We're all the same. We're all rapists. We all deserve to go to Hell and rot there.

I can read every one of her thoughts in the creases of her lips, and hear them every time she sighs or tuts when I look away from her glare. "You've been charged and now we register you in the area. You must stay away from the victim and his family. Stay safe". As she says the last two words, she flicks her eyes at the other one and blushes; she's worried for my welfare but isn't supposed to.

"Get your clothes off. Hurry up". Blondie starts tugging at my top and pulling at my denims at the same time; I pull away.

"Ok. Wait. Let me do it". Crying quietly, I turn to face the wall, wearing only my underwear.

Made to turn left, right, a little more left then right; it takes nine minutes for them to photograph my 14 tattoos and the large hockey scar on my left knee. "That's a nice one", Brunette says, gently touching the large dragon tattoo I have spanning my left ribcage.

"Thank you. It hurt", I reply quietly, and start to cry harder.

"Right. That's you", Blondie says, turning me to face her. "Get dressed and we'll do headshots and fingerprints and put you in a cell. Standard policy". She hates me and I don't blame her. "You go and get the kit ready. Don't forget the mouth swabs", she instructs Brunette. Left alone with the blonde, I feel so ashamed I want to try and explain.

"I didn't mean it to happen. I've not been well. There's stuff I need to say".

"Shut up. You're a sex offender. You're a woman. It's disgusting. There's nothing you can say. Best be quiet".

It hurts having my fingers pressed hard onto the ink then onto what looks like a large photocopying machine. The blonde one's doing it, pressing harder than she needs to and Brunette's pretending not to notice. "Do you want a book to read in the cell? You seem the type", she says, her voice muffled by the large cupboard she's almost disappeared into.

"Yes, please".

"Anything in particular?" She's waving two books at me and smiling. There's a pain in my thumb as it's pressed hard, for a third time; apparently the machine isn't working properly "again".

"Just give me three, please. Am I here overnight?"

"Yes – you're not out until after court tomorrow". She's inside the cupboard again, looking carefully for books for me. The kindness spikes my chest and I want to fall to my knees and shout how sorry and ashamed I am. "Here you go". She's neatly piled three books up and is leaning against the counter. "Swabs next".

It's a bit like a cotton bud being gently scraped against your cheek; not unpleasant, but sitting there smelling slightly of sweat and stale alcohol, greasy hair scraped back by hand, and mouth wide open, this is actually the worst bit. "That's... you... all... done... nearly...just... about", Brunette says, sweeping my mouth with each word like we are at a perfectly normal beauty or dentist appointment.

"Stay sitting there. Last thing is headshots. One to the left. One to the right. One straight on looking here". Blondie's right in front of me now. She holds my face in place to show me the right line to look at. I'm reminded of the last time I had passport photos taken.

※※※※※※※※※※※※※

"I'll pay you back when we get home, Baby". He's cupping my face in his hands. "I can't wait! I need a holiday!" He yells from the bedroom as I hear the scrape of his suitcase being pulled from the top of the wardrobe.

"We don't need to pack yet! It's not for a month!" I laugh, standing in the doorway to the bedroom, leaning with arms crossed against the door. Thrilled he liked the surprise, I'm slowly relaxing from the tension I've felt all day since booking the surprise holiday to Portugal as an anniversary treat for us.

"This is the best bit!" He yells, picking me up and swinging me around.

※※※※※※※※※※※※※

That holiday he sexted three women we met; one wasn't yet 18 and later became my dogsitter. Well, until she decided to ghost me for no apparent reason. Of course, I found out the reason eventually and he denied it. But the pictures she sent me of his penis made a liar of him, yet again.

"Stop moving your head. Sit still". Blonde's saying. A tear falls into my lap and out of nowhere a paper towel appears in my hand.

The cell's not what I expected; it's bare of anything bar a small metal, seatless toilet, and a long blue mat. There are two blankets folded neatly at one end, and what looks like a blue plastic pillow. Nothing to look at. Just four grubby, scratched, graffitied walls and the toilet. No window. Nothing. On the ceiling some professional spray paint reads, "If you're here because of an alcohol problem, get out then get help". I can't bear to look at it, so roll over and wrap myself up in one blanket and use the other to make a softer pillow than the one provided.

"I need to see your face!" A voice yells in the food slot in the cell door. It's one of many welfare visits. Every 30 minutes. Sleep is not an option. Perhaps deliberately. I don't care. I just want to see Phoebe; hold her, sniff her fur, and curl up with her to sleep, more than I think I've wanted anything my whole life.

"Dinner!" A slam, bang and a slide of metal wakes me from a half-sleep. In my dream, I was running and clutching uselessly at the hands and fingers pulling and tugging my clothes. There were flashes of light and a clammer of voices.

"Breakfast!" A deep voice yells, and a kick on the door to make me move up and out of the blankets.

"Ok Ok Ok. Thank you". Disorientated, I stumble towards the hatch and take the cereal bar and the plastic cup of piping hot tea. "Ugh. Sugar. I hate sweet tea". Muttering and unwrapping the bar, anger wraps herself around my neck. "All your own fault", I say to myself.

"Shower, then court", a plump, brown-haired officer says, leading me to the communal bathroom and handing me a small bar of used soap.

"Is there a towel?" I ask the new person who now appears to be in charge of me and the other inmates that I've heard shouting and snoring in the night.

"There's these. Just get on with it". She hands me a bunch of paper towels.

"Ok. Thanks". It's a bit late to care now anyway. It is what it is, and little do I know that the worst is yet to come.

****

Standing in the dock, staring straight ahead, I hold my breath and pray to go deaf and turn to stone, blanking out the next two minutes of my life. My hands are cuffed so I can't put them over my ears, and they are shaking with the tension of utter humiliation.

The public gallery is fuller than I expected; I didn't even know that offences like mine were heard in open court. The shock of around 50 faces all turned to look at me as I was led in is in is nothing in comparison to the audible gasp they all emit as the Court Clerk reads out the reason I'm here.

She reads out my address, a little too loudly or perhaps it just echoes in the terrible silence of the cavernous, windowless, court room. With no window to focus on, and no option but to stare straight ahead, I purse my lips and refuse to show any emotion. Dark wood, dark eyes, and even dark leather seats surround me, and it feels like I'm already in Hell; where these people, every single one of them, think I belong.

The only opportunity I've been given to speak is to reply "yes" to confirm my name. It's not like it is on television. You don't say your plea, your solicitor does this for you; a decision taken down in the cells below the court an hour or so before you're called up. "I recommend Not Guilty for now so we can gather our thoughts and await the evidence from the Criminal Prosecution Service. It's been several weeks since the… erm… event, so of course no DNA; and I can tell you it wasn't Sam who reported the offence. It was his mother, Carolanne Jacobs".

Not making eye contact, I jiggle my knees and pick at the skin on the side of an already-ruined thumbnail. It bleeds a little, so I suck it and remember I used to suck my thumb as a child for comfort; to such an extent that one is slightly smaller than the other, even to this day. This Day. This terrible day.

"Yes, I know. It was my friend, my best friend, who told her". Lauren had her own reasons for it, and I have to accept it. I've waited for this, for the last few days. It was always going to happen. She thinks she has a right to destroy my life and even humiliate Sam. I just need to take it.

"What? No. It was a Kay Larkin who apparently made the call". Pain and shock cocoons me and I start to hyperventilate.

"Kay? But she's my friend! She said she wouldn't say anything". My voice weakens at the end. How disgusting I sound, wanting to have kept my secret safe. Kay's not the issue here; I am.

Hang on. I told Kay, a few months ago, actually! Why hasn't she said anything before?! Surely the fact she sat on this information has some sort of impact on the credibility of her statement?!" Clutching at straws isn't warming my solicitor to me.

"It doesn't say here when you told her about Sam, but it does say she has some text messages between you, so the police are focussing on that right now!

"Yes. There will be some". I'm resigned to this now. Of course, she didn't delete my messages, even though I asked her to. Flooded with relief and trust, I'd wittered on and on about what to do about Sam for a few days after the last Forgivers Club meet. Off-loading everything that had happened, desperate to feel lighter and less alone, Kay had lulled me into a false sense of security and kept every last word, for this very occasion. My lynching.

"Do you know why she would betray you like this?" the solicitor asks, shuffling papers.

"The same reason all women betray each other. Jealousy", I whisper. "She had a thing about her husband leaving her. Recently I've had some issue with Sam's mum and other people in the village; Kay's obviously been influenced and finally joined in. She sees me as a homewrecker. The worst thing ever, to her; worse than... than... well... you know".

That's that then; all my friends have betrayed me, as I betrayed them. My biggest mistake was trusting myself to make a life free of mistakes! I came here broken and I broke everything around me. How the hell am I going to tell Ben? He'll run a mile now; no, ten miles to get away from me.

The solicitor's talking again; "We'll get you up to plead Not Guilty. You'll be signed out and can go home, but there'll be a series of different bail conditions you'll need to comply with.

Obviously not talking to the victim or any of his family members..." The word victim makes me shut my eyes in pain.

I want to put my hands over my ears and shut this all out. "... and you'll be recalled back in around four weeks to change your plea if the evidence is stacked against you. At that stage, I will recommend you plead guilty. But let's cross that bridge when we come to it".

"There must be something you can do?! I didn't hurt him. Force him. Anything like that. Pleading not guilty won't make any difference. I did do it. We did do it". As I say the word "we", his lips purse in distaste.

"He wasn't of legal age. It's not rape as there's no law of "rape" in these instances where the perpetrator is a woman, but it is sexual intercourse with a minor, and that's where we are headed in terms of a conviction. Like I said, wait for the evidence pack and we can talk more then. Be grateful you aren't being remanded; but do consider this is an unusual and extreme case, and the judge assigned may well give you a custodial sentence".

He pushes his chair back and turns swiftly to walk away. I want to scream after him to come back and tell me everything will be ok. I won't go to jail and I won't be murdered when I get home. He disappears around the corner and the cold of the police officer's hands takes me by surprise as she holds my wrists together to cuff them and walks me back to the cell.

"Don't speak to anyone in here. They don't need to know what you did. Safer that way". That explains why I'm in a holding cell alone, and the others are all laughing and chatting together in cells around me. This is it now; I'm a sex offender. I don't cry but I do sit on the bench with my back against the wall and tuck my head inside my jumper for warmth and privacy, so I can stare blindly ahead, bargaining with God and going mad inside with no one to see me.

"Your phone. Your keys. £2.56 in change. A dog poo bag. No, two dog poo bags. A scarf, aaaand yep. That's it. All your stuff. Sign here". The officer pushes a clear plastic bag through the square hole in the metal mesh screen between us. Someone snorts with laughter behind me, but I don't turn around.

"Thank you", I whisper, signing my name and sliding the clipboard back.

"Pen!" The officer barks, as I start to turn away.

" Oh, sorry. Yes". Simply out of habit, I've tucked it behind my ear like I do when I'm at work. The thought of telling Jen - oh God! and Louise - when I get home makes me want to scream. Maybe I won't even get a chance to call them. Carolanne and her flying monkeys will have run riot this last 36 hours.

Feeling sick with fear, I walk as fast as I can to the bus-stop opposite the court, and sit down on the cold metal seat. I immediately start shaking with the cold and shock. Arrested yesterday morning, I wasn't prepared, so haven't got a coat. I hope Phoebe's ok. She's going to be absolutely freaking out. At least I'm going home! Relief makes me want to cry, but it doesn't last long.

I hear her before I see her. Carolanne's driving down the road towards the bus stop tooting her horn and yelling something. "Paedo bitch! Paedo cow!" Over and over. She has a new word for her repertoire now.

A flash of light takes my attention from her, and I realise I'm being photographed. "Go away!" I shout, and fumble for my phone. I stop when I realise there's no one who would come and pick me up, even if I did call them. And the police aren't exactly going to help me.

I start walking, fast, away from the bus stop. "Wait! Lola! Turn around! Take your sunglasses off! Come on, sweetheart!" The journalist is following me. I can hear the clicking and whirring. He's an insect, and his photographer is a lawnmower. I feel hunted.

Turning, I stop, and he smiles at me. A wide, sharky smile. "Leave me alone!" The tears in my throat make the words weaker than they have ever been.

"Come on..." The photographer creeps closer and the journalist flinches; this is his moment. No one else's.

My shoulders feel so heavy. "Please leave me alone..." The photographer starts snapping again. Fuelling each other, I don't matter, as they follow me another few yards as I cry and beg for them to leave me alone.

Out of the corner of my eye, I see Carolanne's car pull up on the other side of the road. She gets out, shuts the door, and puts a roll-up in her mouth, never taking her dead eyes off me. She leans against the car door, and grins.

"She called you?" The whisper seems to have more of an impact on the sharks circling me, than my shouting and crying. The photographer flicks a look at the journalist. In that instant I know I'm right. "She called you? And does Mother of the Fucking Year not actually care about her son? No?! Well, I assume you lot certainly don't! Where you splash me on your pages, you also splash him. She knows that and that's how little he matters to her. She is more obsessed with me, than she loves her own son!" The journalists all look at Carolanne and I feel something like unease. Ah, the penny is dropping!

"The real story, the before, the why and the background to Sam and me, is standing over there. I'm just the scapegoat; her son will suffer more than me in the long run!" Yelling this into the group of pale, unhealthy, unfit cretins who feed on misery, feels pretty good.

Fuelled, I turn and march away to a corner I know leads into a small housing estate. There will be another bus stop there where I can shelter from the rain and think about how the hell I am going to get through the next three years on the Sex Offender Register.

The crowd of vultures has dissipated; perhaps finally realising that there is more to this story than a puffy-faced fool who broke the law and humiliated herself and, even worse, her victim.

Wiping the seat at the other bus stop with my sleeve, a hot tear falls onto the cold metal and my throat tightens in sheer shame. How has it come to this? I had such high hopes of recovering from Jamie and Sharna. Too high, clearly. I don't deserve to be anywhere but the gutter, or perhaps Hell.

Sitting down heavily on the still damp seat, I feel a presence next to me. "It'll all work out as it should. Chin up".

I can't bear to look at the pensioner next to me. I hear him slide closer, and can smell peppermints and lavender. This only makes me sob; the shaking of my entire body feels like it might demolish the bus stop. "There's a tissue for you. I'm sure things aren't all *that* bad? Boy problems? Is there no one who can come and take you home?" The man presses a tissue into my hand, and squeezes my wrist gently. His hands are small, wrinkled, and warm. I think I want to hold them forever.

Then I remember... *Ben.*

Listen to: Dolly Parten and Kenny Rogers – Islands In The Stream

Chapter 18: The Island

The car smells nice; like it's new. There's a faint hum of vanilla and it reminds me of my first boyfriend's car. I adored him; he was my first proper sexual partner but after about a year of my usual neediness, he cheated on me with my younger friend. She was 15 and gave him a blowjob in his car while I slept off a vodka binge a few metres away, in the cottage we shared.

Out of nowhere I want to scratch my own eyes out and peel the skin off my entire body. "Look. You don't need to talk if you don't want to, but I did just pick you up from outside a court and that's a very fetching plastic bag you have there", Ben's not looking at me but he's paler than I remember from the other day. There's a small pulse throbbing in his neck and he's stubbly, like I've not given him enough time to get ready properly. It's after 5pm and a Friday. He was probably chilling out with his first beer or wine of the weekend. Feet up in front of a fire. Music on or maybe a film.

"I'm sorry. I know this is weird. I don't even know where to start or what to say. I'm sorry". Leaning my head against the cold of the car window feels strangely pleasant. It's warm in the car which I think is a BMW or an Audi. It's definitely something fancy. It's immaculate but on the dashboard, I catch sight of a small pink hair bobble. My chest squeezes. Kids? Wife? Girlfriend. Just great. Bloody great.

"It's my daughter's". He's read my mind. "We didn't get around to it yesterday. I'm separated from my wife. Jess. I left her a while ago now. It didn't end well". He looks at me for a reaction, understanding? Or forgiveness? I've plenty of that.

"Why?" If he talks, then I don't have to.

"Long story and not for just now", he says and changes gear as we go uphill. We're near Bridgefell, and I want to get out of the car and run away in the opposite direction.

"Tell me when and I'll stop", he says, slowing down and cruising past the pub. Carolanne's car isn't there and the relief makes me feel physically sick, but it's followed by panic and I'm expecting to see her parked at the Bistro; she's not. She's probably talking to those journalists; there were three of them.

"Just here. It says, 'Have your Cake and Eat it above the door'". I'm already unbuckling my seatbelt; determined to run in, grab Phoebe and a bag, and leave. No, I'm not; I can't. The bail conditions document in my pocket rustles as I open the door. "Shit"

"Shit what?" Ben says, putting the handbrake on. "You look scared to death!" He's holding my arm so tight, it hurts. I don't want him to let go.

"I'm mortified about the court thing and my friends are in there. Well, one of them. The last one left. really".

He opens the door for me and merely says, "You've me as well now. Come on. I'll come with you".

****

Louise is sitting quietly in the corner of the bistro watching us; she's yet to say a word. "Well, you made a right mess of things then, haven't you?" Jen says, while icing a tray of Belgium Buns. She's having one of her "good days" today, although there's a distinct tremor in both hands and her apron is hanging off her now very small and thin frame.

"You could say that, yes". I can't bear to make eye contact with Ben, and I've explained enough to prepare my friends for the oncoming village uproar. Louise uncrosses then crosses her legs again, and lets out an exaggerated sigh and follows it up with an eye-roll just for good measure. She wants me to know she's livid. She's saving all her anger and name-calling for later, when I'm not here. Jen's in for a right earbashing for "taking in a paedophile" and "trusting someone clearly not to be trusted", "a virtual stranger", and "village bike". I can almost hear her.

"I'll take Lola with me, if it makes it easier for your both". It's the first time Ben's spoken, and I'm shocked it's not a similar reaction to Louise. For once, I might actually have found myself a decent bloke.

"I need to stay here and help in the shop. It's a busy time. Jen's not well. I can't just bugger off and hide". I haven't even told Ben that's what I was doing when I turned up here last year. What a bloody mess!

"You can get me through this busy patch, Lola. Stay a few more days and then maybe take this, erm, what was your name again?" Jen's gone pale; she's having one of her moments.

"Ben". I fill in the gaps for her. I flick a look at Ben as I say his name. I've recently started to call him Bear. It suits him.

"Yes. Ben. Ben's offer if things get too much here, or we go back to Portugal. Whichever comes first". Jen's confused now, and spinning left and right looking for the icing spoon that she's still holding. The stress of what I've done, the disappointment, it's making her ill. More ill, each day.

The phone in the office starts to ring and we all jump. "Guess who that is?" Louise strides past me, almost pushing me out of the way. "It's going to be a right shit storm now".

In the end she was right; journalists started calling all hours of the day and night, wanting to know as much as they could about the Stranger who'd arrived to "groom and abuse" the "vulnerable local child" described in the horrendously exaggerated news reports that followed over the next few days.

There were false bad reviews with awful allegations of "rude" staff, and "bad" food that were neither on shift nor even on the menu, which the faceless trolls claimed to have sampled. By day five, Jen was destroyed, and I wasn't far behind her. Louise's thunderous face and nasty comments in my ear every time we were left alone, accelerated; Ben's offer was looking my last and only option for the next few weeks, until my next plea date in court. The bistro had rocks thrown through the front door three times; tiny shards of glass were being found in corners for weeks after my conviction. Sharp, blood-inducing little reminders that, whoever was doing it, wanted us as destroyed as the glass panels they kept shattering.

The final nail in the coffin came from a call about Carolanne's own sentence for chasing me in the street and ongoing stalking. "She was offered a fine of £400 and has cited low income as her reason for not paying it", the clerk's voice is young and cool. They have no idea how this news has shattered the last bit of resolve I have left.

"What do you mean? She runs a pub?! It's not even her first offence against me! Don't you have the list of other times the police were called or went and spoke to her? There should be six or maybe seven before the shouting in the street thing!" My voice is high-pitched and frantic while the clerk's has gone in the opposite direction.

"That's not for us to consider. We were given a report of a woman shouting at another woman in the street. That's what we graded the offence on. That's how it works. If there are other offences or charges, the police have a responsibility to provide it to us. In this case, if you are telling the truth, they didn't".

"Well, that's not good enough! It's been months she's been at it! Months!"

"Well, take it up with the police in your area. We read, grade and report the offences. They are the ones who investigate, charge, and report it to us". The line goes dead. Crying with anger, I call and leave a message for the officer who most often attended when I've reported Carolanne; already expecting the brush off and more buck-passing, I wasn't disappointed.

"It's up to the CPS to request additional information on any accused referred to them. It's not our job to tell them what to sentence someone to", his voice is flat and emotionless, bar a slight tone of boredom.

"You know what she's been doing. You're not protecting me or investigating the crimes, the STALKING, properly. That's your job!"

"Like I said, report any incidents and where there's evidence, we will interview and maybe charge her. That's what we did". Trevenna knows fine well; he knows fine well that Carolanne is out of control, and he's weak and pathetic to be allowing it to happen.

"But you didn't give all the info to the CPS in the first place?! So even with a charge mistakes are being made! Plus, you let her go all these times and didn't tell her not to approach me! That's a mistake, too!" It strikes me that as I report the offences against me, the attending officers aren't recording all the facts. Their boss then chooses to record a more minor offence such as malicious communications or breach of the peace. So when it gets to the CPS, they have bare info and meagre powers to seek a trial. Yes, this has gone beyond mistakes; it's become deliberate neglect of the law. Why though? Ineptitude, laziness... or is she perhaps a police informant?

The officer's still waffling on in his familiar whingeing yet monotone style. "It's not me who decides what she gets charged with. It's a decision taken above me. The desk sergeant on duty makes that decision. In light of recent events, she had her own reasons for the behaviour you say you have experienced".

Rage ignites a fire in my belly, and I lean across the table as though he was in front of me. In desperation to be helped, I'm holding the phone painfully close to my ear. "She was stalking and harassing me for months before she even KNEW about what I did with her son! Months. Do the maths, you idiot!" My eyes fill with tears as the adrenalin of anger pools in my feet and the rush of fear, that no one is stopping my stalker, starts to take root.

"Look. I apologise for losing my rag. Please understand, she is relentless and, to be honest, has always bullied me. I hate that word; it sounds so pathetic and immature..." I put my head on the table and growl in confusion at why this woman is so uncontrollable and determined to ruin my life.

He sighs, then the words I hear are take my breath away. "It's just some tit for tat between some local women, and not really something the police around here are usually drawn into".

Slamming the phone down, I'm now surer than ever that I am being deliberately left to rot and suffer at the hands of Carolanne. Downstairs, I can hear Jen and Louise arguing. Well, more Louise going on and on at Jen about getting rid of me. Every now and then I hear Jen's softer, lower, voice replying, and I can tell she's trying to defend me but not winning.

A few minutes later, there's a light tap at the door; I know exactly what's going to happen next. "Lola. There's someone to see you. Downstairs". Jen's face comes into view and she's even paler and more lined than when I last saw her, this morning.

"What is it? What's happened?" With my chest thudding and a cold sweat already forming, I follow Jen downstairs with Phoebe close behind. She's extra needy with the horrendous atmosphere that seems to be getting thicker and more suffocating by the hour.

Standing in the centre of the bistro, looking a little awkward, are two police officers: no, not police, but it's some sort of dark uniform for sure. Then I see the logo and my breath catches. "No, no, no, no..." I start to whisper. I think I know what's coming.

The female steps forward with her hand outstretched to shake mine, then glances at my feet to Phoebe. My blood runs cold as realisation of what's coming squeezes my heart so tight, it hurts. "No, no, no, no", I babble. I think I'm having a panic attack already, and the woman's not said a word yet.

"We've had an allegation of animal abuse and neglect Miss...". Jen collapses into the chair nearest her, and gasps.

Louise is standing at the till, but looks up to the ceiling in disgust. I think I hear a series of exaggerated tuts. Perhaps, for once, she is backing me up. Albeit in her own special, low empathy, way.

"Neglect? What do you mean?! What type of neglect? Abuse?" The tears come easily, and I start to shake.

"We had someone call us yesterday saying they see you regularly shouting at your dog, and that she is afraid of you. The person also went on to say, they have seen you hit your dog. Down on the beach".

"No, no, no, no! None of that's true! I love my dog. She's my child. *My baby*. Please don't take her!" Falling to the floor, Phoebe's delighted and starts to jump all over me, licking my face and wagging her tail, thrilled at the sudden affection. I close my eyes and put my face in her fur, praying this isn't the last time I get to do this. As usual, she smells of biscuits and my own perfume.

"Can we just take a look at her? And have a chat? Look, let's just pull this back a bit. It's just an allegation right now and... to be honest, this looks like a reasonable place to be living, and the woman refused to leave her name... so we take these types of calls with a big pinch of salt".

Opening my eyes, I watch her as she bends down to my eye level, and begins to examine Phoebe's mouth and ears for any signs of health issues or neglect. Her face is kind; she's older than me. Phoebe jumps up on her back legs to try and get a sneaky lick in. The officer laughs and gently pushes Phoebe down.

"Your dog, she clearly adores you. She's very fit and well, actually!" The officer laughs as Phoebe takes a chance and jumps up again, putting her paws on the woman's knees.

"She is! We are virtually inseparable. Please don't take her. I'm being harassed, stalked, by a woman from here. The call will have been her. I just know it!" The other officer steps forward and appraises Phoebe from a distance. I think perhaps he's in training, or doesn't want to get white doghair on his dark blue uniform.

Wiping my face on my sleeve, I stand up and look at both officers, begging them to believe me and go away empty handed. This is horrendous; all far, far, too far now. "She even tried to take my dog recently. She stole clothes and now I got myself in trouble and did something terrible, by my own stupid mistake, and thinks she has a right to totally ruin my life! She knows Phoebe IS MY life!" Crying again, I'm now sitting next to Jen, who looks like she's going to be sick.

"I understand. We'll leave you in peace now. Phoebe is clearly fine. We get false reports every now and then. In my professional opinion, this was one of those". She steps away from Phoebe and smiles at me as she notes down what she's decided.

"Will you tell the police what happened? If I get them to contact you?"

"Sure. Give them my details and we will give what info we can". She hands me her card and turns to leave. "When people start going to these lengths to hurt you, it's good advice to keep your head down or even leave the area. There's something... evil... about targeting a family pet or a person's job or child, to win some sort of petty war. I see some horrendous things in my job and they too are also done by evil people. Something wrong with them". Visibly upset with the state of Jen and me, and how her time's been manipulated, the officer leaves with nothing more to say.

"See! See how evil that bitch across the street is!" Spinning around I point at Louise, hoping for some sort of sympathy or words of comfort.

"That's good advice she gave you. Leaving...", is all Louise offers before disappearing into the office.

"I don't want to leave you in the lurch, Jen. They, this village, they want me gone. Running away again, disappearing like I'm ashamed, is the last thing I want to do. I'm happy to face the courts, but it's affecting you and your business, and poor Phoebe now. Carolanne's getting what she wanted. For me to have nothing to live for. Today was a close one. You and Phoebe are my closest friends. You're my family!"

"Lola, you have Ben". She stands up and walks away from me towards the counter, then turns. "He's your island in the storm now. I need to support my wife in this, and I think you should go, too".

***Listen to: Meghan Trainor – Like I'm Gonna Lose You*unset**

Chapter 19: Rattling

"Lauren!" Shouting and running across the road, I'm trying to catch up with who I think may be my last friend in this place. Yesterday's horrible shock with the RSPCA officer, and Jen's devastated face as she suggested I pack up and leave, have me angry enough that I'm mistaking the heated, reckless emotion coursing through me for bravery.

"I can't be seen talking to you, even if I wanted to", she says without turning around.

"What do you mean?!" Running ahead of her, I stand firm, so she has to stop and look at me. I am in her way and she can't escape me.

"Lola, you know exactly what I mean. You went with Oliver. Just like I knew you would!" Her face is red, and she's been crying but now, she's livid, not hurt.

"You have no idea, Lauren. No idea at all, but I can tell you, you're wrong. Really wrong". Feeling sick with worry and battling an impending hangover that I absolutely deserve, I hold her arms and refuse to move. "There's stuff you don't know, and Kay's got it wrong, because Carolanne's at the heart of all this. She's evil"

"Stop blaming everyone for your mistakes. You shouldn't have come here. All you've done is ruin lives and cause damage. Not just Sam. *Everyone*. We all want you gone so we can get our lives back!" She pulls her arms away and looks left then right for a gap in the traffic so she can cross the road to get away from me.

"Listen to me, Lauren. I need to talk to you!" My pleading is pointless. She's running across the road crying again, now. I can hear her sobbing and muttering.

"Come near me and I'll kill you and your dog myself!" she yells, once on the other side. Braver now she's three metres away.

"Keep your cheaty sleaze of a boyfriend, Lauren! He's all yours!" I yell back.

She makes a rude gesture and grins madly. I watch as she jogs towards the entrance of the pub, and think I see a movement in the shadows; Carolanne's watched the whole thing. She's loving every minute of this, especially now she has a reason to ruin my life and make me suicidal. She can glory in her victim status, and enjoy the toxic fame that comes with it.

Lauren's right: it is my fault. If I hadn't gone near Sam, at least I'd be the victim; but how long I could have put up with the inept police and her insane harassment, is anyone's guess. "Let's go and pack, Phoebe. It's time to leave. For your safety and then mine. In that order".

****

Over the next few days I pack up what I have, and notify the police and my solicitor that I'm changing address temporarily. "I'll collect you tomorrow, around 10am. Okay?" Ben's been a dream; easy going, helpful and, so far, not interrogating me about what happened or why I found myself in such an horrendous situation. Maybe because he's older or simply just a nice person, either way I don't have the energy to ruin it and be triggered into demanding why he's so nice, not yet.

"Can I use your computer? I'm going to see if there's a reason why that bitch can stampede my life and get away with it over and over again. There's something fishy about that cop and her. The rest of them are just followers and smallminded, judgemental people, scared of the truth. But she, she... she's different and so is he". Babbling on and a little drunk, I know I sound crazy; Ben's not going to put up with my own special recipe of bonkers and intense for long, but fuelled by wine and gin, I'm just going say it. He can bolt if he's not up for letting me stay.

We're sitting on his big gold velvet sofa, by the fire. He gets up, crosses to the dining table, and slides the laptop off. Handing it to me, but not letting go, he makes me look at him. "Lola. Just be careful. You've got enough to deal with, without going rattling cages here and there as well".

I pull the laptop, but he holds tight. "I need to try and make sense of all this. I've nothing else to do!" Pulling it hard, he lets go. Sighing, he leaves the room and I immediately feel terrible. No matter how hard I try, I hurt and / or piss off anyone who seems to give even the smallest damn about me. "Shit".

"You've always been pig-headed and stubborn", my father's voice in my ear. "Never just letting things go. Moving on. Letting sleeping dogs lie", he whispers, on and on. It reminds me of Jamie, all those miles away. Constant gaslighting; telling me that I was paranoid. Demanding I simply accept his version of the truth.

I know there's something wrong in how Carolanne can stalk and harass me, and apparently other people in the small village long before I came here. How she can be so brazen, cocky, and fearless of the police... I type in "police informants" and start to read.

A movement nearby tugs me out of police misconduct, fraud, misuse of police informants and the deep, dark, murky, world I think I've fallen into. "Lola. You're a complete idiot. A stupid person". Ben's sitting on the coffee table and leaning towards me. My heart stops; he's one of them!

"But I think you are also a good person. Too trusting. Naïve even". Relief makes me faint and lose my grip on the laptop, and it slides off my lap. "You did a terrible, foolish thing. I know what that's like. You don't deserve to suffer for the rest of your life. You're going to take your punishment from a court and no one else".

I want to cry with thanks. "Be careful who you target with this police corruption stuff though. Focus on your own case and not Carolanne for now. She's dangerous". Frowning I'm not quite sure what he means.

"You haven't met her, have you? Do you know her?" He sits back and looks away out of the window into the night.

"No. I know *of her* though". His voice is hushed, almost a whisper. "Before I had this house, I was involved in some stuff that you could say wasn't legal".

For some reason, I want to laugh at how politely he's putting his confession. "There's a sort of underbelly to this place. Those of us involved keep our head down. Do what we do and have a sort of code. We don't mess with anyone not involved, and we don't take... the piss". Now I do laugh. This is insane; and I think it's the first time I've heard him swear.

"It's not funny, Lola". He's affronted, and it only makes me laugh more. I think I'm going crazy. What the bloody hell is going on! "I'm not involved anymore but I live a quiet life, never made any real enemies, and had a good reputation. This Carolanne is what you would call a Nutter. A proper one. She's got in bed with the most stupid cop in the area and they have history". He emphasises the last word and I catch on immediately.

"I was right all along then! She's shagging him!" Standing up, I walk to the other side of the room, away from him. I'm angry with him; he's tried to steer me away from the truth to save his own arse. His very rich, comfortable arse!

"Yes. You are right. Sometimes it's not a good thing to be right, though. Not where types like her are involved. She's dangerous because she has no code or boundaries, or even respect for her own son. She's delighted you messed up; it's now her ticket to drive you to Hell and back. Taking him and his own privacy with her, is not on her radar".

"Yeah, well, only if I let her, and I've no intention of rolling over for her. Not anymore". Leaving the room, I think I hear him swear again, under his breath.

****

"I'm going to recommend you plead guilty at the plea hearing next week. Sam has given a police statement and confirmed that you did indeed have sexual intercourse at your flat on the date already given". The solicitor's right. I was going to plead guilty anyway, never any doubt. Carrying the secret's only served to make me ill; and with all the vigilantism and Carolanne's constant harassment, I've lost the will to lie or fight any harder over this.

"Yes. No problem. Can you assure me I won't go to jail? I can't leave my dog". He thinks I'm crazy. Worried about my dog, yet I'm one of the most famous female sex offenders in the UK right now. The media have made sure of that.

"I can never guarantee that, but I would suggest that although it's possible, it's unlikely". The words are a blessing.

"*Thank god.* What do you think I *will* get then? I can't do community service because my name and face have been splashed from here to the moon and back; and I'm already being stalked by his mother and her mad mates". My solicitor sits back and steeples his fingers.

"Let's wait and see. The court won't apply a sentence that's untenable for you, as they need to be firm but fair, and make sure you complete the sentence; so it's in their interests to make it achievable as well as safe for you".

Leaving his office and stepping out into the street, I take a long deep breath and look up at the sky; closing my eyes, I let the cold air slap me hard in the face and hurt my lungs. "It's going to be ok. It's all going to be ok" I whisper over and over, walking towards the bus stop. All that time carrying the secret, when really, I could have started my sentence within days of it happening. It was fear of being killed in jail and losing my baby that rammed my mouth shut. I'm angry with myself, a lot. All that wasted time. All the shame and fear. All for nothing.

"Paedo slut bitch!" A voice shouts, and a flash of black almost knocks me off my feet, as Carolanne's car speeds past.

Her face out the window and a rude gesture then, as usual, she's gone. It's the third time this week she's managed to be somewhere I am, even tens of miles from her pub and my Ben's house.

"Stop fucking following me!" I shout uselessly, at the now empty road.

Sitting in a bus stop, even though I'm headed to the car park to get my car, I know I'm safest here. There's an elderly man next to me and buses going past on a regular basis. I'm having to constantly calculate where I can find a witness, and hang around them or walk near them, ready to have them see or hear Carolanne's almost constant, auditory attacks.

Yesterday it was the hairdressers in Padstow; the day before it was the shop near Ben's house. Now she's exposed herself as the long-term stalker, blighting my life since the spring, Carolanne's escalating. She's actively tracking my every move; making her presence known loudly, and obscenely, no matter who's watching. No matter where I am or what I'm doing; it's as if she's always there.

Running footsteps behind me make my heart stop. Any loud noises, especially car horns and shouting, make me spin on my heels and raise my hands up, as if in defence of whatever attack or confrontation is facing me. The doorbell and the phone both terrify me in equal measure, and I've stopped answering any unexpected communications. Both the house and mobile answer machines have a recorded message explaining I don't answer withheld calls and, if they don't leave a polite, detailed message, they won't be getting a call back.

The recording also explains that if anyone is visiting, they can call or text me from the doorstep to request permission to visit. Ben's bought CCTV cameras and signs, and we have three dotted around the house and made sure one is at the gate to his property. The list of protective measures feels endless but, without them, I am more of a wreck than normal. Whatever normal is. I came here to find it in myself again: that elusive and safe "normal". But it's still hiding from me as I hide from the outside world.

The police are logging every incident, but Carolanne's being what passes for clever, by making sure her acts are short, sharp, and unwitnessed wherever possible. She is always in her car, which enables her to disappear as fast as she appears.

Indeed, she's making sure that no one can identify her but me. Frustration has me short-tempered with Ben, and fear has me rooted to the corner sofa by the window, at Ben's house, watching the road for her car as often as I can be. On bad days, many times a day, I see it drive by several times. It's like she's circling the area, and getting a rush out of imagining me sitting alone at the window, and making sure I feel watched.

****

"She's making you ill, Lola. More ill than you were when you did the thing she hates you for". I look at Ben, and I know he's right.

"Well, she was making my life a fucking misery before she knew about Sam and me!" I snap back. Ben flinches and pushes his chair back so hard he has to stop it falling and clattering to the kitchen floor.

Immediately, I feel bad for being so bad-tempered. My fight or flight responses aren't just reserved for Carolanne and her group of vigilantes; Ben gets it in the neck, far more than he deserves. "Ignore me. I'm sorry, Bear. I didn't sleep very well last night, and my nerves are frayed... as usual". He sits back down and reaches for my right hand; my left is grasping a paintbrush. Carolanne or perhaps one of her mates has painted "Lola is a cow" on the wall by the front door.

We've checked the CCTV and it came up with nothing, but there's a way to get onto the property if a neighbour has left the gate open at the back of their land. Looks like the vandal has put in the effort to watch and wait for the opportunity, then run across the fields, just to do this. The blatant vandalism is almost in double figures now.

"Lola, I think I should sell up. We can go..." I interrupt him with a slap of my other hand on the table.

"No! We aren't going anywhere. No way. Let's face it, look at all the ways and how hard she has looked for me and targeted me! If we moved to the moon, she'd fucking email Mr Moon's secretary and hassle her to make us leave. Then Mr Mars' secretary, then Saturn's PA..." Ben's laughter shuts me up and I smile, although a tear lands on the table in front of me. "I'm trying to joke about it, but we both know I'm right, and that's the saddest thing of all. She wants to run me out of here, make me go, but will madly stalk and harass us wherever we end up. The hypocrisy and warped irony of her obsession... is... I don't know... Is the right word... psychotic?!" Laying my head on the table, I start to cry openly.

"We will do whatever you want. When you're ready, we will go. If you want to stay, we'll stay. With any luck, someone else will rile her and she will target them. She's too lazy to stalk two of you to the same degree!" I feel his hand as it brushes the top of my head.

"Thank you, Bear. I don't know how you cope with all this and put up with my mood swings and nippy-ness".

"Because I love you, Lola. I have done since we met. You know that". He's kneeling beside me now, and I lift my head up to look at him. A rush of acceptance makes me say exactly what he wants to hear, and it's the truth.

"Well, you're stuck with me because I love you too". He flushes with pleasure and my acceptance turns to guilt, quick as a flash. All I ever do is hurt people. "I don't want to do this to you anymore. It's unfair. It doesn't matter how we feel... this situation is knocking us both sick, and it's hardly a happy relationship in the midst of this nightmare. You should go and meet someone else". Ben sighs, stands up, and wordlessly walks from the room.

****

Ben's barely spoken to me these last few days. He's deep in thought, distracted, and even sometimes a little moody with me. That's a new thing; he's always so sweet and laid back.

"Do you know where my pink coat is? That ugly bright-coloured one, that I don't even like?!" I call from the walk-in wardrobe, and stop rummaging to listen for Ben's (almost certain) helpful reply. There's nothing. Stepping back a few feet, I look around the doorway to see where he is. He's standing with his back to me, looking out onto the garden; even from here I can see it's snowing.

"Bear?! Did you hear me? Are you ok?" I'm walking towards him barefoot and he doesn't turn around, even when I embrace him from behind. It always surprises me how tall and broad he is; I might as well try and hug a phone box. "Earth to Bear? Earth to Bear? Transmission attempt number two!" Trying to sound upbeat, hoping to soften him up and end the strange coldness between us, I squeeze tighter and force a smile. Ben's muscles loosen a little and I think I'm making headway, thawing him out.

"Transmission received, Captain. Pink Coat sighted in spare bedroom, on the bed. You may attempt a recovery mission. Over and out".

Now I do smile, properly; we always had fun. Flattered each other with the same sense of humour, and refusal to take anything too seriously. Well, until Carolanne started.

"Bear, I'm going to try harder. I don't want to meet anyone else, and I don't want you to meet anyone else. I'm sorry for what I said. That hurt you. It was cruel and it was untrue". My honesty and apology surprised even me, and Ben turns around and stoops the foot-and-a-half difference in height between us to kiss me.

"It's hard, I know. Come on, let's go and land our ship and have a cuddle before you go to your appointment with the solicitor. Try not to think about tomorrow and the sentencing. I think we have a spare 11 minutes…" He smiles and his eyes light up in mischief. There's the Ben I know.

"Go on, then. That gives me a spare six minutes after to find a weird hat to wear, as part of today's disguise".

Dead on 10 minutes later, we're back looking for the rest of my outfit; I've started to change what I wear when I leave the house. Instinct tells me she knows to look for my usual big grey puffa coat and pink bobble-hat. I've been making it too easy for her to spot me, now the streets and roads are a little quieter. I don't take my car as often, as then she follows me in hers; I refuse to buy a new car every week!

Ben's sitting on the edge of the bed, with various hats and scarves on his lap. He's laughing at me, and his big shoulders shake with the effort to suppress them. He knows this is serious even if it is bonkers.

I'm knee deep in clothes and have my back to him, but can almost feel his mirth. "Bear, I mean it! Help me find a scarf and hat I've either not worn recently or at all!" Turning around and throwing a yellow woollen headband at him, I carry on breathlessly searching and talking, far too fast. This signals my anxiety level is high, again. "I think she'd kill me if she had the chance, and we've already agreed she has the means to get away with it". Ben's sat on the end of the bed watching me.

"I've been thinking about that…" The tone of his voice makes me turn sharply.

"Go on. Let's hear it".

There's easily ten seconds of silence as Ben gathers the right words, then he sighs, looks down at his feet and, as if making a decision, closes his eyes and shakes his head. "No. It's a mad idea. Extreme. Silly. I wouldn't do that, not even for you". He mutters this but it's clear, by his lack of eye contact, his idea was a bad one.

"Good. I don't want to know. Keep that zipped!" I walk over to him and kiss him hard, to stop him blurting out his idea.

****

"Someone sent this to my ex-wife". Ben's handing me his phone. The screen's lit up with a screenshot and it takes me a few seconds to work out what it is. "I don't understand. She lives abroad? She's been gone for ages!". Ben poured me a large red wine as soon as I walked into the kitchen 40 minutes ago. Taking my hat and coat off, I'd picked up on a strange mood but, tired and ready for a bath, I'd put it down to a long day and all the worry finally catching up with him.

"It's a paedophile hunter site. With your name, and the address of your flat". Ben's voice catches on the P-word as I wince and close my eyes.

"I don't even know what that is? What is it?" Handing the phone back, I don't want to read it. "Explain it to me. I can't bear to look at it!"

"It's a sort of online poster or page thing. There are loads of them. Mostly men, of course, but your one has had loads of hits and a few hundred shares already". I start to cry and so does he. "My wife is *livid*. She's stopping me seeing my daughter because you're here in the house and we are seeing each other. She's furious and disgusted and well, you can imagine what she said. She said a woman sent the screenshot to her with the words, 'Thought you should know what your husband is doing and who he is doing'". You can guess who the woman was, Lola. Your old mate Carolanne. One of the shares on the page is someone called Lauren. You had a pal with that name, didn't you?" I watch as he gets up and leaves the room, and my heart clenches even tighter, as I watch Phoebe trot after him.

Things were relatively quiet after the webpage surfaced; most likely because Carolanne was basking in the pain she was causing, and the relative notoriety meant she had her grubby hands full. I'd reported the page to the police and shown how it linked to the village and people I knew, but I was fobbed off with some story about how difficult it was to investigate anything internet-based like this.

****

"Are you ready?" Ben's voice through the noise of the shower.

"10 minutes!" I call and almost choke on the water as it streams in my mouth. It's here; the sentencing date. I've dreaded yet looked forward to it. It's difficult to explain. Fear and relief jumbled together; a sense that today is the end of one stage and after my sentencing will be the start of another. I'd said much the same to Ben in bed last night and he'd smiled for the first time in days "it's a good job you're an optimist" he'd said as he kissed me. "I don't think another human being could have put up with everything you have in the last few months".

"Yeah well…. I deserve some of it. I know that. It's easier to deal with when it's my fault. It's the stuff that is out of my control and totally uncalled for that makes me… sick and angry. Maybe after the sentencing she will stop? Or at least then I can be seen as admitting what I did so, be more deserving of peace? People can't stalk and harass someone who's admitted their crime, can they? Someone decent enough to admit it and try to serve the sentence?" Ben's arms squeezed tighter, but he didn't say anymore and that unnerved me, just a little.

Outside the court, a row of journalists are standing in a cluster; bored, listless, and smoking cigarettes. Heads together, hunched from the rain, means they haven't seen me yet. The urge to stop walking, turn around and go back to the car and then Ben's lovely, secluded house overwhelms me, and I stumble a little. His hand squeezes mine then he tugs me forward. "Keep going. Stay strong. Don't speak or look at anyone. Stare ahead. Don't smile or grimace; no expressions as these bastards like to take one of your face in motion. To make you look as ugly or crazy as possible".

I put my sunglasses on, squeeze his hand and walk forward but it's difficult; I want to run over to these so-called-journalists and ask them why, if they are so good at writing, none of it is ever the truth or even, particularly clever.

"Lola! Lola! Let us see your face. Take your sunglasses off! Go on! Give us a smile". All their voices clammer together and we walk faster. Once inside the court building, every looks at us; aware we were the ones the paparazzi were waiting for. They'd clung to the fact I was almost 20 years older than Sam and a young-looking blonde; gloried in the storyline using words like Rape and Romp. Both words polar opposites but still selling papers in equal measure. How can a "Rapist" actually "Romp" with anyone? Of any age?

Which one am I? Some sort of seductress who "romps"? Or a rapist? Or am I someone in between. "In between" doesn't sell papers. In between is usually closer to the truth. In between is the grey area of the law and of justice that less intelligent people (paid in those sectors) fear. There's a difference between not being able to legally consent, and what people see as "rape".

Rape emits images of violence, scars, blood, tears, and life-long trauma. It's not a grey area yet it's applied in many none-violent events of sexual contact, where indeed alcohol, drugs or even age were a defining factor.

I was raped when I was just 17. I had a boyfriend who I adored. I just got myself in a silly, drunken situation. I was spiked by two men, barely known to me. Both men had girlfriends. Both decided that, once my friend left me at their caravan, I was fair game. There was no blood. Some bite shaped bruises on my breasts. No violence. I was passed out for most of it. I have flashbacks. But "rapist"? or "Rape?"... I'm not sure. Legally yes, psychologically... not as much as you would think.

This is all coming up, out of the stinking, long hidden soil of my mind, as I walk past groups of people staring at me. People there just to catch a sight of me. Over and over I think about what I did and how it came to this. The word rapist makes me want to tear the flesh from my face and scream that it's not me. It's not what happened. In law it is but between Sam and me? In our heads, it did not.

"It's going to be over in a matter of hours. You'll be home by lunchtime. Don't worry", Ben said as my name was called out and I entered the court-room to be sentenced. Admittedly, walking past the public gallery and feeling all those eyes on me again, a thought that maybe I wouldn't be going home to a bed, my Phoebe and freedom jumped inside my skull. The fear felt overwhelming as the judge read out their decision. "Three years community pay-back order". Not knowing what it really meant, I looked at my solicitor; he nodded so slightly and so fast no one else but me saw it. I knew then, it was as ok as we could have hoped.

In the car on the way home, I made a promise to myself. If Carolanne would leave me alone now, and let me run my sentence, I wouldn't keep pushing for answers as to why she, so far, hadn't seen a court herself. I repeated this to Ben as we spun into his drive-way and he squeezed my hand with four words "seems fair to me".

Listen to: Linda Ronstadt and James Taylor – I Think It's Gonna Work Out Fine

Chapter 20: A Hiding

The whisper of something touches the back of my leg; I left the house quickly this morning to go on a morning run. Just before sun-up, it was crisp and duck-egg blue but not as cold as you'd expect for late December. A few days after my sentencing, I'd started venturing out and Phoebe was delighted.

I'm panting and breathless but pleased with my running time; 38 minutes for the 10k I just ran. Music on and pushing myself to beat my record, I'd missed the man and woman following me as I walked the last few hundred yards up the hill from the cliff path I'd just run.

Clipping Phoebe back on her lead and tugging the earbuds out, I feel the brush of the woman's skirt on my leg and then her sweater on my arm. Why is she so close to me? Irritated, I turn quickly to face her. "Are you ok?" The words blow out of my mouth, as I'm still out of puff.

"I know who you are!" she hisses in my face, and spittle lands on the tip of my nose. "You're going to Hell", she carries on. Something touches my hand and, looking down, I see it's a card, like a playing card but with a picture of Jesus on it. "You're going to Hell", she repeats and steps back, smiling. She has the strangest face; a sort of long, lined face and, although she's smiling, her eyes are nasty.

Her hair is dyed a dark red and styled in a 1980s mullet. I take all these details in for some reason. The man behind her is bald, short and stocky, and looks a little unsure. He has a backpack on, and I watch as he leans forward and takes the woman's arm; they are together. Fear ripples through me and

I look left then right but, apart from a few tourists now standing watching, there's no rescue or safety of note here.

"And you think with language like that, you're not going to Hell?" I reply, stepping back. "Following me. Coming for me. You think you're good people?"

"You rape children!" she shouts, and I flinch. Hearing a gasp behind me, I realise one of the tourists has stepped closer for a better look.

"Did you hear that? Hear her?!" I say to them. They step away again.

"Filthy rapist. Our friend Carolanne told us about you". The bald man is speaking now, but still doesn't look particularly confident in his role here.

"Tell that mad cow to come for me herself. I've no idea who you are, or what you think you're doing, but she isn't doing this for her son! She's been stalking and harassing me for months!" Both of her minions frown in unison. "She's evil. Don't do her dirty work for her!" I shout ,and run as fast as I can.

* * * * * * * * * * * * * *

"I've cautioned the woman, but we don't know who the man is". The police officer's talking. "You cautioned her? For THAT?! And what about the link to Carolanne?! How did they know what I look like and to follow me like that?! It's sick and crazy. I'm frightened!"

"It was the man we can't identify who said that, Lola. Not the woman". He sighs and I hate him.

"I want to make a complaint. A formal complaint". The officer sighs and gives me the details on how to make a formal complaint. "Enough is enough"! I yell, before slamming the phone down. "Fuuuuuuuck!"

For the next few weeks, I don't leave the house again. "You need to think about getting a job, Lola. Even just a small job. Something basic. I've plenty of money but you need stimulus.

Anything at all". Ben's stroking my hair, and desperate for me to be "normal" or as normal as he thinks I should be.

"You don't understand. Wherever I go. Whatever I do. She's there, or the people who pander to her are there. I'm going to rot away to nothing, and she's going to dance – no piss! – on my grave!" Ben stops stroking my hair and gets off the sofa; I think I've made an indentation of my own small (and getting smaller) body these last few months. "Don't lose patience with me. Please. Ok, I'll try something. I used to write a bit when I was younger. I've been thinking about doing a recipe book. What do you think?"

Ben stops by the door. "I think that has just made my week. Get on with it then!" His smile makes me feel like the sun just came out.

"I'm a miserable cow but I'm a resilient cow", I call after him as he goes downstairs.

"Get on with it then!" he repeats then laughs.

"Maybe I should", I whisper to Phoebe, as she wanders in to see what all the raised voices and laughter's about.

For the next few weeks, I write and write and occasionally leave the house. Ben comes and goes and takes Phoebe with him. She's rarely getting walked as much as she likes, but he's a godsend and she's madly in love with him. I'm close to the edge of that abyss, too. As stupid as it would be.

Emails have been pinging all day, and I've resisted the urge to open them. With a mixture of excitement and trepidation, I keep eyeing up the laptop as though it were a scorpion, and I were laid flat out, tied to wooden stakes, deep in the Mexican desert. Jeez, writing really is for me?! Maybe I should try crime fiction rather than cookery books!

Flicking a look at Ben, I see he's nodded off on the other sofa.

"I'm afraid we can't take your book concept any further". Ok, I can try a different one. "It's not what we're looking for", the other one a few days later reads. "There's no market for this", the next one says. A tingling pins and needles sense of doom creeps over the carpet towards me as I'm hunched over the laptop. I've been foolish; I've gone public with my desire to have a book published. Overconfident and knowledgeable in marketing, I threw the idea out on my business networking site to my 8000 followers; most of whom know my past but are interested in my work anyway.

"There've been rumours. Calls. A woman harassing publishers and platforms interested in your work". The direct message hits me in the jaw, yet I'm not shocked. Is it normal to be shocked but not FEEL it?

"Please ignore her. She's insane. It's been months and months, and will go on years and years. Please don't listen to her. I'm happy to explain what happened and live with it and do my sentence, but I need to earn. To live", I reply and sag with relief when the agent replies with "We are looking into it. Hang tight".

An hour later and I'm in the local pub, alone. Unable to bear telling Ben what's still going on, I've snuck out. A sixth sense told me to leave Phoebe at home. "Another please. Thank you", waving the tequila glass at the barman and smiling; I know I have to leave soon. A woman in a peach top is now going around the pub whispering in ears, pointing at me.

I'm tipsy but not drunk. Going home wasn't an option earlier; I don't do running away anymore. Plus, it's a quiet area and if I leave the pub, she will come after me. Undoubtedly, I am safer here. Watching Peach Top now though, she's rallying troops and, even sober, I'm unsure if I can outrun this giant 80 kilo bag of spanners.

Giving her a thumbs up and grinning, I tip back the tequila and start to spin on my stool. A flash and she's in front of me. "Rapist. That's what you are. Sam's my nephew. Rapist!" Then she spits in my face and headbutts me. Peach Top just spat in my face and headbutted me. Ok, that's different. I'm used to scratchy cats and hair grabbers; not headbutters and spittle.

Automatically I reach out and grab her hair where it's most bunched; a poor excuse of a ponytail, and simply latch on. Not even remotely fazed that the left side of my face is tingling, nor that a strange woman is flailing and hurling herself at me, and screeching like a dog that found a squirrel. I hold her head at my silly long arm's length and stay on my seat until three men untangle her. It's odd how I think this is normal.

Of course it isn't. I have spittle on my face and my left eye is swelling by the second. Frankly, in this oddly awful context, I'm delighted I didn't come close to leaving or falling from my high bar stool. "Shall we order another?" I say to my new friend, and smile.

The bar staff were quite young, and one was new. I didn't know him. Sweet, dumpy, and very gay, he looked at me like I just fell out of a Care Bear's arse and yelled *Bonjour tout le monde*! Really, I just asked for another Tequila and, of course, he laughed. This was a small bar in a relatively quiet part of town, and I've sat in the same seat, for maybe three weeks, and had started to get to know people.

The woman with "electrocuted toaster dyed black hair" always wearing the too-small leather jacket. The guy with the toupee who smiled at everyone, and always had change for the jukebox as long as you played Elton John's "Rocket Man". Lastly, not to forget the ex-NHS midwife who was in the bar from 11.45am every day. She sips a rum and diet coke, and only leaves the pub to buy sandwiches to eat for her dinner. Her daughter died of adult SAD.

I made it my business to speak to people. Get to know them. Spend time. I wasn't below, or above, anyone.

As I walk towards the toilets, I think about how unfair this is. It should be Sam hating me or hurting me; he's the person I hurt, not these relative strangers. I reach up to feel my eye again, to make sure it's not bleeding.

"Sore? Let's get you some ice and go to the loo". A voice behind me. It's one of the girls from the bar.

"Louise... I'm ok. Honestly". She's already holding up an ice-pack.

"Shut up. I'm finished now anyway. Come on. Lay it on. Then we can go home. To be honest, I'm tired". My eye is throbbing now and the urge to close it is getting stronger with each pulse of pain.

"Ok. Have you got a cig?! I'm trying not to smoke but fuck it". Louise laughs at me and we get our things and start to head outside.

I really need to head home. My new friend is tired and now seems rather drunk. Fag in hand, she's leaning against an Audi and I'm waiting for the car alarm to go off. "Come on, you stay near me, let's walk". I'm taking Louise's hand and she's floppy and laughing at my silly sensibleness.

"Stay a bit. We can go in a bit", she slurs. I lean back again against the wall and take a breath of patience, and want to laugh because I know this is going to be a hilarious short walk home.

"Oi, you leave my fucking mate alone!" Why Louise is shouting I have no idea; it takes me a few beats to pick up on it. A group of people; just colours, hats, and hair, are headed in our direction. I am slow on the uptake. Then I'm on the pavement and my friend is screaming.

Strangely, it's not a painful experience. All the more frightening because I know near my ribs and shoulders is my head, my brain. People don't die from kicks to the hips, legs, and ribs. That's honestly what I'm thinking, as I curl up then kick back out myself, as if a spring inside my gut has been let loose.

Not my head! Not my brain! is what I keep thinking. Silly to you, but next time you get attacked in the dark and are on the ground, the thing you will most fear is brain damage or facial disfiguration. I promise you that.

I have on daft high heels and 90s wet-look leggings, and a beaded jacket; none of this is made for street fighting. But I am made to defend myself. My mother made sure that I was built to *fight back*. I start grabbing at the hands either side of me and swearing like I've woken up. *Woken up angry.* I pull my legs back and kick out; hard. And kick again. I feel that I've finally hit flesh, then hear a cry of pain.

Satisfied, I kick again and pull again. Then again. Sensing one of them has gone, the one to my right. She's fallen or been pulled by someone. Spidery, I buck and am on my feet, arms raised and head down. "She's seen us. Go. Go. Go", someone shouts and in seconds the street is deserted.

A few hours later, I'm clutching a slightly-bent cigarette and crying in shock. "Can I ask if you have purple highlights in your hair?" the male officer asks.

"Why? How do you know?" He's not in my home. He's where it happened.

"We found a patch of skin with hair near the gutter where your friend's earring was". He sounds young and oddly freaked out.

"Yes", I say, and want to laugh. It's all so disgusting and evil. I imagine how I tied my hair up in Heidi plaits. Mainly because I couldn't be bothered washing it. Apparently, attackers find it easier to pull the hair from the head if it's neatly tied up.

Raising my hand to my head, I slowly stroke my hair and feel nothing different, so my heart relaxes. Then I let my fingers gently wander up my head, a little further, nearer to my crown, right at the top. It stings and feels hot and is smooth. Nothing. No hair. Just a sore, burnt bit. "Take a picture! Take a picture!" I yell at Ben. He winces and looks like he might cry.

"Are you sure? Maybe best to leave it a bit…"

"Take the fucking picture", I hiss, and a fat tear falls on my lap where my leggings are torn. I start to take my shoes off; one is broken, and one is covered in scuffs. How I got home, I don't know.

"Ok. But please don't get angry", Ben, and I hear the click. Then another one. A gasp. He's looking at the picture. "Lola…"

I turn and grab the phone. He was right to gasp. I echo it; a 50p-sized, no bigger, space on my scalp where my hair used to be. I was never blessed with big thick hair. Never the girl with long locks of waves. Never ever the mermaid or the princess in the school play. This, above the harm and the blows and the bruises across my body is, to me, the worst. I drop the phone. Ben me, and I cry.

I certainly got a hiding, although not enough to kill me. Well, not that time.

Listen to: Toto – *Africa*

Chapter 21: She's Dead

"I need to see you". The text is simple and not exactly grovelling but, to be honest, it's how I'm rolling right now. Lauren is the softest of the lot and, for a fact, Carolanne's enjoying letting her be manipulated by the group. Her misery before Christmas, when we parted ways, was deeply upsetting and back then I was selfish; focused on my own survival in the court case, and not hers in the hellish relationship she has with Oliver. I feel like I owe her the truth, whether she likes it or not.

"I don't want to see you", she replies fast; yes, she does. She's missing me. I know she is. To not ignore the message and not block me, means something. Of course it does.

"If I agree to answer all your questions and tell you things about Oliver that you don't know... will you meet me then?" She snaps the bait off the hook and I'm thrilled. I'd rather have no friends and be honest, than have no friends and regret not giving them the truth.

"Go on, then. Let's hear it". Lauren's sitting on a bench at the beach, overlooking the sea. She's thinner than I remember and my chest hurts looking at her. She reminds me of me, before.

"Oliver's a dark person Lauren. Darker than you could ever imagine". The opening sentence doesn't even make her flinch. "He tried to rape me". Then she flinches.

"Don't lie, Lola. All you do is lie", but her voice has no real power; she's just saying what she thinks she should say.

"He did. I didn't tell you partly because I had no chance, and partly because I didn't think you'd believe me. He's your everything and if I said he had a second head you'd deny it, even if he was standing there waving the damn' thing about, and laughing at you out of both mouths!" There's a flicker of a smile then. I wonder if she's finally ended it. "Where is he now? Are you done?"

Her hands tighten on her lap. "I think so. Yes. Things haven't been right this last winter. Since you left". She says this and refuses to look at me, and I'm not surprised. She was never bad like them; just addicted and afraid and frightened.

"Look. Let's just strip this back, Lauren. I did not, ever, have any interest in Oliver. I know he did in me and you saw it. Other people saw it. His behaviour and your own fears… fed what happened between you and me. We've both dated Narcissists now. I understand. I think maybe you do too?" She turns to look at me, and I see a hollowed-out, sad, deeply-entrenched person. I want desperately to fix this for her. I wouldn't wish dating a Narcissist on anyone.

"What are you going to do now? You know Oliver always comes looking for you when he's ready". She laughs loudly and it's like lightening. The cracking shattering sound scares me.

"Not this time he won't. Carolanne saw to that."

"Do you think Kay would consider talking? To trying to work our way through this? We were all friends once and, to be honest, I'm struggling. I can't work. I can't sleep. I can't breathe for the next drama and just want to get through this".

Lauren's face softens "You can try. She's not been around the last few days. The pub's been closed and, to be honest, no real way or reason for us all to meet up".

"The pub's closed? What do you mean?" My heart flutters and immediately I'm worried about Sam, where he is. How he is. If he's safe. Keeping this to myself I don't dare voice the concerns. "If the pub's closed, where the hell is Cray Cray Carolanne?"

Lauren laughs, again so brittle. "Who knows? Who cares? She made all our lives a misery. I think Sam got lumped off to a family member along the coast, or maybe up north. But don't say to anyone I told you". She pulls her hand away and stands up. "I need to go anyway. Just in case she's watching. You know how it is".

No longer keeping secrets from Ben, I decide to trust him finally with all the reasons I left home and came here. I don't hold back on how suicidal I've been nor how I've drunk too much and even, at times, relied on drugs to block it out. I tell him about Oliver and Kay and Lauren and even Rob; enough details that I no longer feel afraid of being my true self. If he really cares for me, then he will stand by me.

"It's time for me to be honest with you, Lola". Ben's voice shatters my resolve. "I'm going to go. Whatever you have to say is only going to ruin this. This is how these conversations go". He tugs me back down to sit at the kitchen table. "Not this conversation". Now he has my attention.

"Ok. Go on".

"I just want a quiet life. A quiet life with you and Phoebe. I don't even like dogs. She likes me though". Phoebe walks out of the kitchen and out of sight.

"Not that much just now". Ben snorts at my awfully-timed joke.

"Lola. I mean it. We can fix this and have peace. I want you to stay here. I love you". The words I've heard a hundred times from probably a hundred liars mean nothing.

"Yeah. Ok. They all say that. Let me finish making dinner".

He slams his glass on the table. "Fucking listen to me!" and I sit straight back down in shock. "For once in your life, listen!"

I did listen. I finally just relaxed into what Ben was offering me. I gave up in all the right ways. So frightened for so long, I realised that I wasn't doing myself any favours by pushing away the few people who were prepared to stand by me.

"Lauren says she spoke to you the other day. I hear you want to talk to me too?" The message from Kay is a splash of cold water and yet it's welcome.

"Yes. Please. Just to clear the air. Please, Kay". She blue ticks the reply. "Oh, I hope she meets me". Ben rolls over and pulls the blankets off my legs and reveals Phoebe curled up there. She looks up, ears back and glares at me. "Not my fault this time!" I whisper, and pull the duvet back. "Come on Kay. You know and knew so much more about me than anyone. I forgive you for going to the police. It was the right thing to do". She blue ticks again and I wonder if she's so mortified to have sat on the info then shared it, she's unsure how to tackle a meeting with me of any kind.

"Let me get back to you", she finally replies then blocks me. Oh well, better than nothing.

Things seem almost peaceful but, in all honesty, I'm on edge. To have peace after all these months... years of noise and worry and pain, isn't easy. Then the calls start, numbers withheld again. "Don't answer them", Ben says, grabbing my hand as I reach for the hand-set.

"Oi! What's up with you?!" He looks at me, but it's not surprise on his face; it's fear. I've never seen him afraid before; even his lips are pale, and I think I see stress lines I've not noticed before. "What's wrong?!" I'm afraid that it's finally happened. He's got fed up with this whole thing. Fed up with me. Met someone else. "Who's on the phone, Ben? Tell me. You're scaring me now". My voice wobbles. This is my worst nightmare. I can't cope with this alone, and losing him would be unimaginable. In only six months or so, he's become my rock, my safe place, my future. Everything. I took my time feeling love for him but, now, I think I've messed up. Yet again.

"Nothing and no one, Lola. Nothing for you to worry about anyway. Just business..." Before I can stop him, he leaves the room.

* * * * * * * * * * * * * *

"She's dead!" The top line of the text is short and to the point, although still doesn't make sense.

"Who? What do you mean?" I type back, and the message on WhatsApp blue ticks immediately. Lauren's got some serious gossip if she's sitting online, waiting to talk to me. Either that, or Oliver's with her and not at work. It's probably a celeb again. Not a surprise seeing how the media like to target people.

My phone starts ringing with the WhatsApp call, and dread starts to pool in my feet up through my body in a matter of seconds.

"Go on then. Give me the good news. Carolanne's topped herself with all the guilt of years and years ruining people's lives. Especially Sam's!". I'm trying to cover up the worry of what this is about, with dark humour. Lauren takes a breath in.

"You are psychic. I swear to god, Lola". She whispers, and I can hear her voice is thick with crying. I recognise her upset-voice. It's almost always about Oliver, though. I've heard it plenty of times since we became friends last year. Wow. It's actually a year. I open my mouth to tell her that our friendship-anniversary is next week, but she babbles over me, loudly now. Panicked. "Let me finish. Please! I need to get this out. I'm freaking out!" She's yelling. This is all happening too fast. "It's Carolanne who's dead. On the beach. Dead for a good few days, I heard. Ohmigod! The police are all over the village. They want me to go see them later today!"

"Why do you need to go see them?! She's topped herself. Surely!" My throat is tight with fear, but something like relief tickles my chest. "She hurt a lot of people, a lot of times, over a lot of years, Lauren..." I'm trying to calm her down and make her feel a little better. "She's finally woken up and, like the rest of us with bad mistakes in our past, has considered ending it all. Only difference is, she went and did it. She always did have big balls". Lauren's sobbing and that scares me somewhat. Why is she in such a state?!

"Lola, there are rumours she was a police informant. Because of that, oh, what's the word..." I can hear her gasping and hiccupping in panic. "Foul play! Yes, that's the word, well two words. Foul play! They know she most likely had enemies but as a drugs informant... well... Bridgefell isn't safe for one. Not at all..."

"I don't know what you're talking about, Lauren. But get yourself together. Anyone would think you finished her off! I know you well enough to know you're too much of a wimp though!" I try to make her laugh again and fail spectacularly. I have to hold the phone away from my ear as she wails as if in pain. "Lauren!" I shout, hoping to boss her into calming down. "I was just joking!"

"No, Lola. You don't get it. It's Oliver. Oliver's not been home for a few days. He went out on a... job... .a fishing job... yes, one of those. And he's not been home or in contact!" Here come the hiccups again.

"Well, that's how he is, Lauren. He's likely off with some lassie from down the coast. Sorry to say it, but you signed up for that!"

Lauren stops wailing and goes quiet immediately, and I regret my brutal response to her fear. "Lola. Oliver's a drug trafficker".

Listen to: Nathaniel Rateliff and The Night Sweats – S.O.B

Chapter 22: Guilty Party

"So, you're telling me that Carolanne was murdered by drug traffickers because she's an informant? She's been feeding info about local drug dealers and stuff to the police?! Are you out of your tiny, but beautiful *mind*?!" Lauren's sniffling into a tissue, and wrapped up in her striped dressing gown like a hobo. An hour ago, I found out that Bridgefell isn't as *perfect* as it seems. And the townspeople are *a long way* from it.

"That's exactly what I'm saying!" Lauren yells in my face. "Oliver's killed her! I just know it. It's why he's nowhere to be seen. He's laying low. Hiding out. On the run!" Her Channel 5 police knowledge has improved, and I can't help but smile.

"Lauren. Come on! He's a creep. A letch. He tried to... pretty much... force himself on me after spiking me, and there's a trail of broken hearts and broken beds from here to Penzance but...Murder?! Nah." Lauren looks up at me and all I see is fear. She's not convinced. "It's more likely me that the cops will want to speak to. I've been getting withheld calls all day. But I'm not answering. Fat chance. I've been on my own a lot these last few days as Ben's been at some conference thingy in London". The thought that I may well not have an alibi for whenever Carolanne went to sleep with the fishes thuds painfully. I'd not even considered that. "Shit! Do you think they'll think it was me?!"

Lauren drops the tissue in her lap and puts her hand over her mouth. "What did you say about spiking? Just then. Go back a bit!" In my haste to try and reassure her and help her organise her thoughts, I've slipped up. I never had any intention of telling her the full story of Bonfire Night.

"Look. I didn't want to tell you. It's nothing. Let's just park that. Discuss it another time. Deal with one crisis at a time!" I'm standing up and moving away from her. If I were Lauren, I'd hit me for, yet again, keeping another dangerous secret from her.

"Lola. Tell me what happened!" She's behind me, but I can hear in her voice that her teeth are gritted; this is her special, cold, angry, voice that usually is reserved for confrontations with Oliver.

"Ok, Lauren". Sighing, I drop my head and close my eyes. "Ok, but only If you promise not to chuck me in the sea, like Carolanne! Yes, then I'll tell you. And most important of all, promise me you won't cancel the murder but replace it with a plan to lose the plot! It's a good job Oliver's off on one of his shag-fests. I think maybe he's safer that way…"

****

Lauren actually took it better than I thought she would. Immeasurably better, actually. I've just hugged and kissed her goodbye, and I'm now heading home. My head's whirling but I feel a strange sense of peace, blended with hope. I don't feel guilty for it. Not one bit. Because of Carolanne, I've considered killing myself more times than I care to admit. Even Ben has no idea of the dark places my thoughts have gone. Especially since she contacted his wife.

"That's me home Lola xxx". The text lights my screen up and happiness surges through me. Bear's home and we can wade through this fresh drama together. At the end of the day, the police have to have some good officers! I haven't seen Carolanne since a few days before my sentencing. In the end it will be proven it was an accident, or a pissed of drug dealer from Columbia or something. It won't have been Oliver and, who knows, she may well have actually killed herself and not been murdered. It's early days. "She was only found a few hours ago… well, this morning", I mutter, parking the car at the gate and unlocking the padlock we recently put on it.

"Hi!" Ben's practically running towards me. He looks happy. That makes a change. The front door's open, he'd been sitting at the living room window watching for me. "Have you heard the news!?" Yes, he's excited and not even trying to hide his joy at all our problems – well... most of them, being washed up on the shore this morning.

"Are we bad people for being glad?!" I ask, after he releases me from the usual bearhug.

"No. Not one bit. You and me, yes, we... have had almost *months* of hell, Lola. She's evil. Well, she was evil. Now she's gone there will be plenty of people secretly, and openly, pleased. Trust me on that". Ben's getting in my car and gesturing for me to get in, so he can drive it up to the house.

"I'll walk this wee bit, Bear. Need a bit of fresh air, to be honest". His face falls but not for long, as he quickly remembers that we now have our lives back.

Something feels odd, out of place... off, about all this. He's the happiest I've seen in months. He's been away. He has... connections..." Fuck! Fuck! No *no no no no!* He's responsible for Carolanne's death! He's not seen his kids since she contacted his wife. He knows I was considering leaving him, so he could get some semblance of peace, as well as his kids back. Either he's done it, or got someone else to.

I start to shake with shock and fear and, for the first time since I found out she was dead, Carolanne has me terrified. All I can think of is my lovely, kind, Bear in jail. At his age, he will probably die there. 25 years is life, I think.

Walking towards where he's now standing, on the steps to the house that has been my sanctuary since all this started, all I can think of is protecting him. How, is a different matter.

****

"Forgivers meeting tonight". Kay's texted me, just as I stepped out of the shower. I've left Ben downstairs, singing along to the radio in the kitchen as he washes up tonight's dinner dishes. I've barely eaten anything. I couldn't. He didn't notice though, and every time he smiled or laughed or said anything funny, I just felt more and more ill.

"I'm not up to it tonight Kay. Thank you for letting me know though", I reply, sitting on the bed and my hair dripping onto the screen, as though I'm crying.

"You have to come. We need to talk about what's happened", she replies, fast. I don't have the energy to go, but I've got an idea.

"Who else is coming?"

"The usual group" her reply is simple, but it confirms my plan.

"Ok. I'll be there. Make sure Lauren comes too. She's in a right state".

****

"I'll drive you, if you like. That way we can maybe get a drink at The Cockleshell on the way home. I might even stretch to some Champagne". Ben embraces me, and I hear him inhale; he loves smelling my hair, especially after I've been swimming. "My little mermaid", he murmurs, and leans back to look at me. Terror tightens its fist around my heart, and I fight the urge to cry and tell him my plan.

"Ok. You drive me. I don't feel very well actually".

"Cool. You go and get your stuff. No need for a disguise now!" He laughs and walks out of the kitchen to look for his car keys. I drop my head and swallow a scream. I know where he keeps his keys. He never loses them. I know how he likes his breakfast. How he can secretly dance and sing really well. I know he wants to get married, maybe even have a baby with me. I know his favourite song is Elton John and Kiki Dee's *Don't Go Breaking My Heart*". I know everything about him. Worst of all, I know he would kill for me and rot in jail for me.

It's dark, freezing cold, and a typical February evening. Ben's still singing along to the radio, while I silently watch the shapes and shadows of familiar trees and houses blur past. "Don't wait for me. Just leave, once we get there, Bear. Ok?!"

"No! We're going for a drink after! I've a hankering for that cider. The one that's called something to do with a snake or a cobra or something". It's a running joke that we can never remember the name of it, and the memory of us both scouring supermarket after supermarket muttering suggested, ridiculous names, for the best cider in Cornwall, makes my head hurt.

"Ok. Well, go for a drive or something. Don't sit in the car park. I'd feel weird inside, at the meeting, knowing you're just outside".

"No probs! About an hour?!" He turns and smiles widely at me. He looks younger.

"Ok", I whisper and lean over to kiss him. It's the last time I will.

Ben pulls into the car park of the hall and waves at Lauren. She's illuminated in the headlights and looks like a zombie. "She looks rough", Ben chuckles and I wince.

"She'll be fine after the meeting. We always are". Opening the door, I pull away as he tries to kiss me again, and he frowns then shrugs.

"See you in a bit!" He calls, and starts to pull away. The urge to chase after the car, tell him my plan, and listen to him talk me out of it, is overwhelming. But I don't.

"Glad you're here", I whisper to Lauren as we trudge up the steps towards the open door. I can hear muttering and whispering. The urgent clammering of surprise and panic.

"Let's get this over with. Hear everyone's theories and worries, and get home" Lauren says, walking into the brightly-lit room. Everyone stops talking and our footsteps echo in the overly-warm hall. A numbness creeps over me, replacing shock and fear, as I see the police officer who's let me down *every single time* I've reported my stalker.

"That's everyone here. Let's get started". Kay is chair for this meeting. She's pale and looks like she's lost weight. Carolanne was a close friend... well, *sort of friend,* for a long time; she must be hurting, even though Carolanne caused her pain in the past.

"Are you ok?" I lean over and whisper. She stares straight ahead and won't look at me.

To my right is Lauren, opposite her is an empty chair. Officer Trevenna is to Kay's left. The toilet flushes and, as if in slow motion, Robert and Oliver walk in, one after the other. They look tired and tense. Robert pulls a chair up, next to the one Oliver's now seating himself in. I flick a look at Lauren but she's grey with shock, and staring at Oliver in utter fear.

"Can we get started, please?" Kay's agitated and seems in a hurry. Even though I'm terrified of what comes after this meeting, I'm concerned that it feels like it's *different*. Like we are here for a different reason, other than to simply confess how we feel about Carolanne's death.

The door bangs and we all turn at the same time. I have to twist in my seat as my back was to the entrance to the hall. It's Ben. He's striding in, holding out my phone. "You forgot your phone Lola...". He's not noticed the strange atmosphere yet, but as he takes his eyes off me, I see him pale as he notices who has come to the meeting. "Well, this isn't weird!" He tries to cut the silence with sarcasm, but it only serves to make Kay flinch and close her eyes.

"You're welcome to join us. She had her sights on you for long enough. You must have something you can share about how you feel or what you are thinking now she's gone..." Kay's looking at Ben expectantly.

"Sure. Beats sitting in the car waiting for her Ladyship!" Ben's pulling a chair from across the room and the scraping sound makes me squeeze the plastic arms of my seat so tight it hurts. This isn't supposed to be happening. It's not going to plan. He can't be here.

Trevenna coughs, and we all look at him like he's just started tapdancing naked. "It's me who requested this meeting. It's the best way to get you all together and have a bit of a… chat… about what's happened". Oliver frowns and folds his arms. This is his tell. It shows that he's worried.

"Can I go first?" I butt in, and the police officer looks at me and reddens. Taking in a quick sharp breath, I open the door to Hell. "It was me. I did it. She deserved it". Oliver gasps and looks at me. Kay makes a strange squeal of horror. Lauren lets out a sob and covers her face with her hands. Robert crosses his legs, and looks up at the ceiling. Worst of all, Ben stands up. He's *furious*.

"Lola, what the fuck are you doing? Shut the fuck up!" Oh, he's livid alright!

"Look. You all know what she did to me. To us!" Ben makes a gesture as though he may place his hands over my mouth, to silence me. Then drops down to sit heavily on his chair again. Tears start to choke me, as he puts his head in his hands. Bear knows me well enough to sense a rant coming. "That woman – no, that *creature*, had no place on this earth. Each of us here has felt her wrath. Been targeted. Had part or all of our lives ruined by her. I just had enough and… well… I hit her on the head and shoved her off the pier. Ben was away at a thing, and I was on my own. I had the perfect opportunity".

Lying like this is oddly easy. I've fantasised about getting rid of her a hundred times.

"No, it was me. I did it". I shoot around in my chair to look at Ben, who's now sat poker-straight and talking like he's reading a script. "I haven't been at a conference. I've been staying in a hotel down the road. I waited for the right moment and followed Carolanne up and along the cliffs, and shoved her off. She was ruining my life because Lola… well… she is *my life*". His face crumples and the last few words are lost in his hands as he hides his face behind them. But I hear him clearly enough.

"He's lying. It was me. The bitch was informing on me and my mates. We're going down for murder instead of drugs. Might as well. These days it's the same amount of time and, frankly, what she did to Lauren, taunting her with my stupid bloody cheating… she deserved it. It was easy. I knew she was informing on us. We've suspected for a while". He gestures to Robert who tips his chair back and nods.

Robert looks completely at ease. "It's true. That mad bitch made mine and Natalie's life miserable when it suited her. I've watched her torture Lola, who… I have feelings for…" Robert's looking at Ben, and a flash of fear crosses his face. "But she's happy with Ben. Well, *was happy* when Carolanne left her alone. Which wasn't often, by all accounts". Robert nods at Ben, who nods back. They've agreed between themselves what's right and has been right all along; Ben and I belong together.

What the bloody hell is going on? I can't speak. My mouth's dry.

"Well, you lot are all liars. This is supposed to be a place of truth and honesty!" Kay shouts. "It was me. I've never got over what she did to my marriage all those years ago. Sleeping with my husband. He was the one who recruited her as an informant, and she loved the power of sleeping with a cop. A cop who was the love of my life! Once he died, she moved onto this one here. Snake in the grass she was". Kay's puce with rage. There's not a tear in sight. She's glaring at Trevenna, who has the good grace to look at his feet, and shift from side to side in shame.

There are a few beats of silence and a few of us in the circle are breathing heavily. "You're all wrong. It was me. It's a big operation. She's blown it sky high, over and over again". We all look up at Officer Trevenna in unison, but he stares straight ahead; refusing to look at any of us.

"She's been a nightmare to handle. Sleeping with whoever she likes. Exchanging info with whoever she likes. Being her handler has been a baptism of fire over and over again. Why the hell I fell for her only God knows! Then she started fucking about with a cop in Vice. Carolanne was nothing but trouble". Exhausted at his confession, he looks for a chair and spots one a few feet away, up against the wall. Speechless, we watch him almost stagger over to it and sit down heavily.

"Yeah? So she was a bugger to work with. So what! You're not going to murder someone for that! I don't believe you!" I yell, and he flinches and closes his eyes, and starts speaking again. But this time more quietly, although we can still hear him. "She threatened to ruin my career, tell my wife about us. Blow 10 years of work apart. Destroy me. I've seen her destroy Lola here, and I've heard what she's done to other people".

"How d'you do it then? Go on". Robert's leaning forward and has his hands on his knees. He jerks his chin up defiantly, but I see a twinkle of mischief; he's enjoying this.

" I smothered her in bed, carried her body to the cliffs, and threw her off. The world is a better place without Carolanne. Fact". Trevenna sits back in the chair and bangs his head on the wall; Robert smiles but quickly hides it behind his hand, feigning a gasp of shock at Carolanne's awful demise.

Someone starts to laugh. As if in slow motion, we all turn to look at where the sound's coming from. It's Lauren. She's shaking with the power of her trademark laugh; eyes shut, she laughs and breathes in, then does it over and over again. I see tears start to fall down her cheeks. They make her grey leggings look like they have freckles.

"You lot are all telling such massive porkies!" Lauren's struggling to speak but Trevenna's eye twitches at the mention of pork. "No offence, officer!" Lauren cries and starts howling with laughter again. Oliver's mouth flickers and he purses his lips. I think he wants to laugh, too. This must be a dream; one of the weird ones I was having when they put me on stronger antidepressants and betablockers last year.

"I killed Carolanne", she continued. "Miserable old cow she was. I've watched her make so many people unhappy. Suicidal. I thought I might as well help her on her way to Hell!" Robert snorts and starts to giggle, then it grows to a laugh. Next to me, Ben joins in. Then Kay. My mouth drops open in surprise as Trevenna's guffaw finishes the circle off.

"Why are you all laughing?! What the hell is going on!" The urge to cry takes hold. "I don't get it! Shut up!" Slapping my knees in frustration only serves to make them all laugh louder. Ben's even started wheezing with the pressure of laughing too much and breathing too little!

"Someone better tell Lola what's going on. It's time she got her life back". Lauren stands up and walks over to where all the bags and coats are in a pile by the stage. Now what?!

"I'll read it. It came to me, so it's my letter to read". She's pulled an envelope out of her bag and opens it. Ben puts his hand on my knee, and I look at him. He's smiling.

"Just let her explain, Lola. It's a letter from Sam".

Frowning, I look towards Lauren who's sitting on the stage. Her little legs are dangling, and she looks perfectly relaxed. Is everyone on drugs?! That would make sense! "Hi everyone". She starts to read, and Sam's face swims into view. I think I can hear his voice.

"My mum wasn't a nice person. Not even to me. She's done some awful, cruel things and almost always to people I liked and cared for. When she went mental over the thing with Lola, she went too far. The worst I've ever known her. She made what happened so much worse. Everyone knew about it, used horrible words, and knew who I was and who Lola was, within a day of Mum finding out. She called my school and the papers before she even called the police. I hated what she did to Lola and what she was doing to Oliver, Robert, Officer Trevenna, and even Ben.

"She wanted me to go for a walk on the cliffs to Boscastle with her. The day that Lola had her sentencing. She was hyped up and nasty, worse than usual. We got to the bench by the lighthouse and she told me she'd been to the court to watch. She told me she was the one who had been calling the journalists and that she was the one who had told Lola's horrible ex and his horrible ex, where Lola was. Where she worked. Everything. She told me that as a group, they have all been part of Lola's stalking and harassment. She told me Ben had called her and told her she was to stop, or Lola was going to leave him. She laughed at that bit and almost fell off the cliff.

"In that moment, I realised how easy it could be if she just fell. Fell away and we all got our lives and futures back. She stepped towards me and started saying how she had packed my bags and bought me a train ticket to Redruth. To join the Army. I told her I didn't want to go. That I wanted to go to Uni in Germany and study photography".

Struggling to read the letter openly, Lauren's voice catches, and I realise she loves Sam like a son. I get up to go to her, but Ben pulls me back. "Let her finish Lola", he whispers.

Lauren takes a breath and wipes her eyes with the sleeve of her jumper , and starts reading again. "... Mum grabbed me and started trying to pull me back along the path to go home. She said I was to leave that night. I tried to pull back and away from her. Told her I was going to stay with Lauren and Oliver then leave to go to Germany as soon as I could. She turned and started screaming in my face. I can't even remember what she said now, she was incoherent with rage. I pulled my hand hard and she lost her balance and just fell, backwards off the cliff".

I look around the group, but no-one looks surprised. *They knew about the letter*. They planned this. If they all confess, no one gets caught. This show is a huge apology to me; for how they've treated me, and allowed Carolanne to torture me. And it's the best way to protect Sam. The innocent in all of this. The *only* innocent.

Lauren's hand is shaking, and the letter is quivering like a leaf in the wind. She seems to wake out of a trance, swallows and uses her other hand, to hold the letter more firmly. "... so, now you know. I've spoken to Kay and she's going to arrange a Forgivers Club meeting and you can all do what is right. Finally. Don't worry about me. I was always going to leave and follow my own path. Mum just refused to listen. It's not Lola's fault what happened and really none of you meant to hurt anyone. Some of you are just stupid". Lauren looks at Oliver and he blushes. "Like Oliver and Robert", she continues and Ben snorts. "PC Plod will help tie up all the loose ends. It's about time he did his job properly". Lauren purses her lips and looks at the ceiling. I can see she's trying not to laugh again. "I'll send you a postcard. Maybe one with one of my bestselling photographs on it. Sam"

"Well, he's a bright little shit, isn't he?! Runs in the family, I must say!" Robert is rubbing his hands together and smiling at each of us in turn.

"Looks like things are going to more settled around here", Kay announces as she stands up.

"Yep. I'll sort things at my end. Sort out some way to quieten the investigation down. It's likely that Carolanne's death will be ruled as suicide but if it gets sticky, we can meet up again, and I'll take confessions from you all, more formally. That will confuse and exhaust my sergeant who's as eager as I am to shut this down and move on to... proper crimes. Sam had a good idea". The police officer is walking past me and putting his hat on.

"Told you the kid was savvy!" Robert yells and nudges Oliver.

I think my eyes are going to fall out of my head, roll across the floor and settle up against the stage where Lauren's still sitting. "I don't know what to say. Thank you". I'm telling the truth; I really have no idea what to say. This has been the weirdest, nicest, bestest 20 minutes of my life.

"What're the chances you'll get your range of cookery books out now?!" Kay embraces me and grins. She looks less lined, less worried than I've ever seen her. "You deserve to get your life back. Pay your dues. Serve your sentence in relative peace. It's only right. No one is above the law, and certainly not Carolanne".

"I never want to hear her name again!" Robert says as he pushes Oliver along, towards the door.

"Me, either!" Lauren scurries behind them and wraps her arms around Oliver's waist. He looks at me and mouths the words, "I'm sorry".

And, actually, I think he really is.

Epilogue

"I think we can call Lola up now! Are we ready for her?!" The photographer's spinning left and right looking for me, but I'm trying to enjoy the moment, observing the guests all happily milling around and talking, for as long as possible.

Ben stands head and shoulders above them, I can't miss him, and I feel a surge of love for the big bear of a man who's seen me through almost four years of hard work, patience, and self-evaluation. His eyes alight on me and he cocks his head in a silent question of why I'm standing in the shadows of the garden, just watching everyone. Then I see him realise that I'm just absorbing every second, and storing it my memory with as much detail as possible.

He gestures to the photographer and points in my direction, giving my location away. I shake my head but wink at him and ready a smile for the man taking the pictures at the launch of my third cookery book . "Ah! There she is!" The photographer walks towards me and raises the camera up, to catch me half in the sunlight and half hidden by the huge cluster of yellow roses, Golden Celebration. We planted them the day after Carolanne's body was found. I take a sip of champagne and close my eyes at the lovely scent the roses are giving off. They've grown and got brighter and stronger. Just like I have, these last few years.

"That's a good one!" The photographer yells back at Ben. Ben gives him a thumbs-up and winks at me. I raise my glass to him and smile.

Listen to: Kygo & Whitney Houston – Higher Love

Afterword

In my experience, The System designed to teach us what we did was wrong, and rehabilitate us, is flawed beyond measure and actually, with weaker offenders, will simply "train" them to hate themselves, give up on life and reoffend out of sheer frustration, and lack of genuine support. I rehabilitated myself, at huge cost, where The System was warped and delivered so badly, that it was going to break me and harm me forever.

We are all one decision away from being involved in the Criminal Justice System. A bad relationship. Getting too drunk. Arguing with someone too intensely. Sending a sexual message or picture. Messaging or calling a person who cheated on you with your partner and being angry, or threatening them. Bullying or trolling someone on-line... the list goes on. These are just some of the hundreds and thousands of emotionally-driven poor choices that people make every day. These are all steppingstones to ending up exactly where I did, and many more before me did, and many more in future will. Remember that.

Be kind to each other. Be honest with yourself. Make the world better by saying something nice not judgemental, or *maybe* even campaigning for better justice systems and social care systems, like I do.

About the Author, L.W. Hawksby

The Boring Bit

Hello, Book Lovers! My name is Lucy Haughey and I write as L.W. Hawksby for now. Raised on the Hebridean Island of Mull, by my Eco-Tourism Entrepreneur parents, I came to live in Glasgow in my late teens for a wider choice of careers. Attracted to the idea of helping people via educational endeavours such as training and public speaking, I worked and volunteered during the day and studied at night to gain three Diplomas in Mental Health & Social Care.

What followed was a varied career in the Charity Sector involving work with Breast Cancer Awareness Projects, Steiner Schools, Employability, Debt Prevention, and Preventing Homelessness. But my career fell away as, in my late 20s and early 30s, I began to make some poor relationship choices and became caught up in a cycle of abuse at the hands of both friends and partners. Sadly, by 2016 I was mentally ill and deemed unemployable due to three criminal convictions.

Chasing the "Holy Grail" of Recovery, I followed a gut instinct to write my story down and caught the writing bug! I now focus on writing books that explore criminal behaviour in those I call "Dangerous Normal People" (the title of my first book about Narcissistic Abuse). I want to help people understand and avoid similar bad paths to mine. Like me, few people choose to end up in the Criminal Justice "machine", and my writing and speaking work will highlight how and why, *wherever possible.*

The Nosey Bit

When I'm not writing (which isn't often!) I am found in my kitchen on the window seat, reading a book or sketching while guzzling horrendously strong black coffee. I can also be spotted pottering in my garden enjoying the sunshine (yes, folks, it does happen in Scotland!) with a Gin & Lychee cocktail. I am a serious foodie and have won a few cookery and recipe competitions. I cook and bake at least once a day for My Family. I am blessed to have three lovely children and three brilliant Staffordshire Bull Terriers. When the mood takes me, I am also rather partial to writing poetry and sketching illustrations, of insects and plants mostly.

This year I invested in a large Garden Shed which shall become a year-round "Creatives' Retreat" for my children and I to enjoy together. When the weather is too wacky, we shall retire to "The Inn @ The Lobster & Gin". This is our tiny, hidden, Tiki-Bar that I created in our walk-in hall cupboard last year.

The Spooky Bit

As a Dark Empath, Cancer Decan 2, "1980 Golden Monkey", with rare A Neg Blood, I can't help but be fascinated by the Paranormal and associated Theology. I am unashamedly a weird, wild, and wistful creature who reads Tarot Cards with decent skill when money's on the table! Not to mention that Ancient History and Mythology videos are my go-to YouTube faves! Well, that's when I'm not brushing up my knowledge of The Dark Tetrad and Attachment Disorders!

If you feel you could review and rate this book, please do! Thank you in advance.

If you are interested in reading my other books, you can find them by searching for them alongside my author name, L.W Hawksby.

Title: Dangerous Normal People. Understanding Casanova Psychopaths & The Narcissistic Virus.

Release date: September 2019.

What readers are saying

"Probably the most important and relevant book on the market today, covering and bringing alive a whole range of extremely important subject matter that, up until now, has had a habit of being swept under the carpet"

"I found it very educational and I recommend it to professionals as well as any other readers, as it is a real life account of how a Narc operates. It is a compelling book which helped me identify some red-flags to look out for"

"This is a terrific book, which not only charts the author's own personal experiences, but engages and enlightens on the subject matter"

Title: The Notch

Release Date: September 2020

What readers are saying:

"Absolutely Amazing, couldn't put it down. Will definitely be reading this again"

"Loved this book. Chilling read"

"Eerily familiar and exacting descriptions of the craziness, fog, zero-self-worth and numbness you feel in an abusive relationship"

"Clever Interweaving of complex characters with a hint of paranormal"

I try to produce a book every 9 to 12 months, so keep an eye on my social media accounts as these are my expected 2021 and 2022 releases! "CrazyMaker", "Pretty Girls Gone" and "Echo's Revenge".

You can find me on YouTube under L.W Hawksby where I produce educational videos on the topics explored in my books. I also tweet as @LeonoraTheLion and record podcasts on AnchorFM (also linked to Spotify) as "The Narcissist Hunter".

Once again thank you so much for showing an interest in my books and associated abuse prevention work!

Lucy"

For more info on me as an Author and my future projects, go to www.thenarcissisthunter.co.uk

www.ingramcontent.com/pod-product-compliance
Lightning Source LLC
LaVergne TN
LVHW011346080426
835511LV00005B/153